Chasing Normal

Dedicated to Harry – love beyond words

To friends and family – shoulder to shoulder

And to Slater Walker – truly inspirational and courageous

First published 2022, Revised 2025

Copyright © Jo Rothwell 2022
Illustrations © Bryce Rothwell
Copyright © Illustrations Rothwell Publishing 2022

All rights reserved. No part of this book may be reproduced or transmitted in any form by any means, electronic or mechanical, including photocopying, recording or by any information storage or retrieval system, without prior permission in writing from the author.

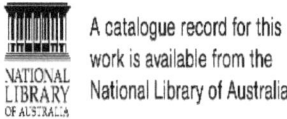

A catalogue record for this work is available from the National Library of Australia

ISBN: 978-0-9944430-4-5

Published by Rothwell Publishing

www.rothwellpublishing.com

Victoria, Australia

Chasing Normal

Balancing the ups and downs of life and cancer

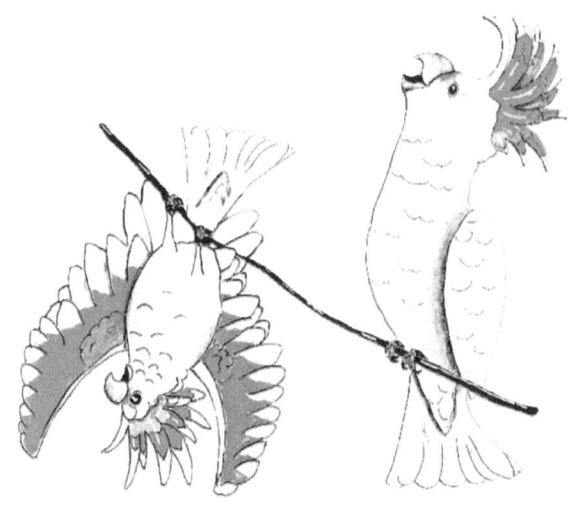

A Memoir by Jo Rothwell

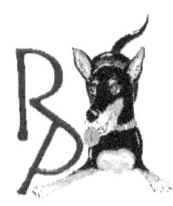

Our lives are better left to chance,
I could have missed the pain,
but I'da have to miss the dance.

Tony Arata
Sung by Garth Brooks

THE PREAMBLE BIT…

I will scream from the mountaintop that cancer will not define me, yet here I am writing about it. Forgive the irony…or not.

There are not many words in the English language that appear to conjure up such trepidation and fear as the word *'cancer'*. Until the age of forty-eight, I was smugly unaffected by the power of this word. Of course, I knew what it meant and had observed its rage from afar, but I was not prepared for the impact of its fury and its command for attention that was about to be unleashed.

This book is simply an account of my experiences, thoughts, hopes and emotions that have been connected to my life with cancer for well over a decade. You may notice contradictions in thoughts and feelings or perhaps simply a growth in understanding and acceptance, leading us to where we are today.

I have no doubt that overall, it will be deemed that my story is my cancer story. However, I hope it is considered more than that. I have included an account from '*Wednesdays with Harry*' between every 'cancer' chapter. *(Please note that they are not in chronological order)*

A few years ago, I started a diary-type narrative of times spent with my son Harry. It was important to me to create enduring memories. And, in the future, if I am not here, hopefully, he will overlook remembering me as the one nagging him to tidy his room, but rather the one who provided laughter, enjoyment and meaningful moments. It seemed essential to compile these memories into written form, perhaps as a keepsake for Harry or perhaps as an outlet for my own need to build words into sentences. Either way, they are intentionally light-hearted and showcase indulgent exaggerations and my personal sense of humour.

I fully realise that some readers may question why I have alternated the seriousness of cancer with the whimsical Wednesdays chapters and perhaps become frustrated with this structure. If this is the case, then you have truly come along for the rollercoaster ride that is my dealings with cancer. It is, in fact, the whole point of this book. One day, I am laughing with Harry, and the next, I am confronted with concerns. The insight is intentional.

Of course, I hope my cancer ramblings create thought-provoking awareness, but honestly, I hope the Wednesdays chapters shine brighter and are valued more. They are the essence of my life and are what gives me strength, laughter and purpose. They are the hero chapters because they put cancer in its place by denying its very existence. Their presence stomps on cancer's power and represents life without intrusion.

To quote Viktor E. Frankl, 'When we are no longer able to change a situation, we are challenged to change ourselves.'

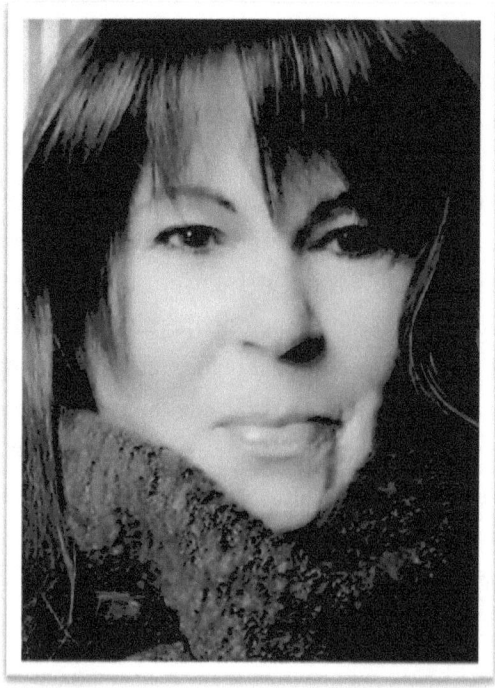

Contents:

The Bit You Need to Read First	1
Reality Bites	3
Wednesdays With Harry... In Art We Trust	7
Up in the Air	11
Wednesdays With Harry... Flat Pack Pandemonium	14
Off With Her Breast!	17
Wednesdays With Harry... Pandemically Speaking	22
Reactions – Under and Over	25
Wednesdays With Harry... True Blue	28
Chemo Extremo	32
Wednesdays With Harry... Dear Mum	37
Hair Today, Gone Tomorrow	40
Wednesdays With Harry... Whistler's Mother	45
Hypnosis	48
Wednesdays With Harry... Warren Brown	52
To Say or Not to Say	55
Wednesdays With Harry... The Buzz Word	58
Hazchem	60
Wednesdays With Harry... Redwoods	64
What About Me?	67
Wednesdays With Harry... Anzac Day	69
Headspace Hero	71
Wednesdays With Harry... Splitting Hairs	74
The Clinic	77
Wednesdays With Harry... Danny Frawley	80
Game, Set...Thyroid	83

Wednesdays With Harry… French Impressionism	88
Living in Limbo	91
Wednesdays With Harry… Cloudy Cosmos	94
In The Pink	97
Wednesdays With Harry… Organising Chaos	103
Thoughts From Close By	105
Wednesdays With Harry… Mountain Ash	110
Metastatic Monday	113
Wednesdays With Harry… Snow Regrets	116
Sideways Effects	119
Wednesdays With Harry… Great Ocean Road	124
R.I.P. Rebecca Wilson	127
Wednesdays With Harry… Triple Antarctic Blast	129
Hypothetical Crisis	132
Wednesdays With Harry…Streets With No Name	134
Art Therapy	136
Wednesdays With Harry…Hold the Phone	140
Appraising the Fundraising	143
Wednesdays With Harry…Paint By Numbers	146
Trial and Error	149
Wednesdays With Harry… Grumpy Old Woman	153
Live to Flight Another Day	155
Wednesdays With Harry…Happy 21st	157
Tired	160
Wednesdays With Harry…Cinematic Joy	162
Oncology Angels	165
Wednesdays With Harry… A Walk Back In Time	167
Faces of Fear	170
Wednesdays With Harry… Rone Empire	176
Casualties of Cancer	179

Wednesdays With Harry… Street Sounds	181
Family	183
Wednesdays With Harry… Bollards	193
Pain Paranoia	196
Wednesdays With Harry… Magical Mystery Tour	198
Riding High in April, Shot Down in May	200
Wednesdays With Harry…God Save the Queen	204
Biggest Morning Tea	206
Wednesdays With Harry… Princes Pier	208
Liver Mets	211
Wednesdays With Harry… Great Expectations	214
Purpose	217
Wednesdays With Harry… Golf	220
Nanette	222
Wednesdays With Harry… Mulligan	224
Dear Harry	227
Wednesdays With Harry…Honour the Memories	230
Them's Fightin' Words	232
Wednesdays With Harry…Aftermath	233
Debbie	235
Wednesdays With Harry…Graduation	238
Tomorrow Never Dies	240

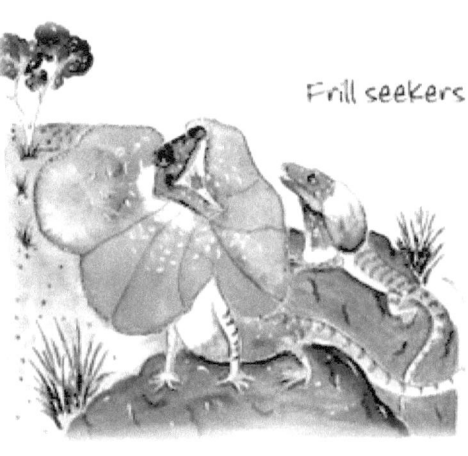

Frill seekers

THE BIT YOU NEED TO READ FIRST

I began writing this book when we were living with the very real threat of Covid-19. It spun the world on its head, and we were forced to proceed with caution. For many, the pandemic introduced physical and mental health issues, perhaps for the first time. My own initiation into a medically provoked upheaval began many years ago…

I live a modest life in the incredibly picturesque Yarra Valley, Victoria, Australia. I dearly love my two golden retrievers and son Harry, most likely not in that order. I am old enough to have spent my twenties exploring the world without fear and young enough to still remember most of it.

I am quite determined not to define myself by circumstance or situation; however, I wish to tell you what is currently sitting close by. I have breast cancer. Not the type that is grieved, treated, survived and hope restored. I have the kind that wants to play a nefarious game. Mortality challenged to stamp its reality when I learnt the cancer had spread. It has wandered off from its original source and constantly attempts to lure me into its power and to fall into a chasm of fear. Prognosis is stage four and incurable.

It began in 2011, when those around me suddenly began to tread lightly, words were lost, and the manual for behaviour was incomplete. Since then, I have become a student in the cancer classroom. I acknowledge its rebellious nature but understand that it is a part of me. Lessons learnt include resilience, acceptance, purpose, distraction, adaptability, perspective and a master class in humour.

Clearly, I don't have it all sorted, as I absolutely feel the grips of mortality as a scary and lonely place. It is owned entirely by yourself, and no one can buy into it. Needless to say, everyone travels their own path.

But my life is not about cancer or about fear. My life is about hope and purpose, adventure and laughter, curiosity and insight, learning and understanding, and love.

To counteract cancer's chaos...I chase normal.

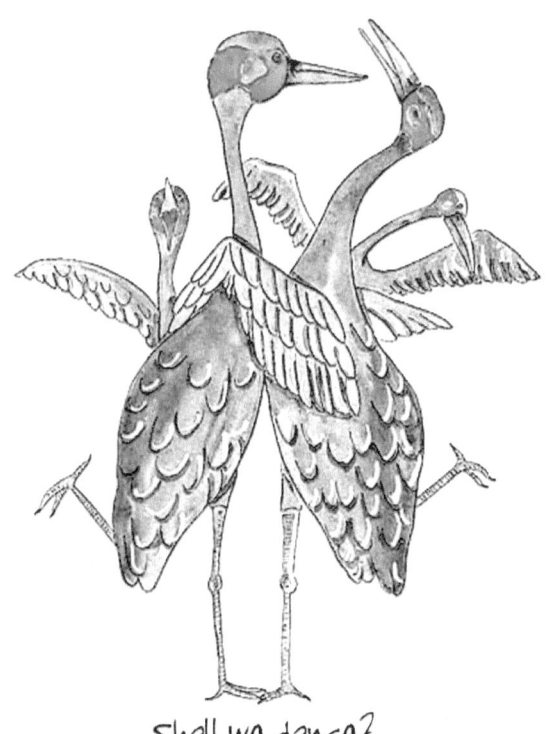

Shall we dance?

REALITY BITES

If you asked me to name a significant date in history, February 23rd, 2011, would be it. Not a date that marks a natural disaster, the declaration of war, the discovery of penicillin, or walking on the moon. In fact, it is not a date of tremendous historical importance to the general populace. But for my own personal history, it is by far the most significant.

On the morning of February 23rd 2011, I drove myself to the breast surgeon's office to receive my test results. I was consumed with the thought that my life may never be the same. I remember waiting to turn at the crossroads of Corduroy Road and Warburton Highway on the outskirts of Yarra Junction when a wave of reality crashed upon me and halted my journey. I suddenly couldn't breathe. Anxiety had taken hold and was clinging on, determined to mess with my mind. Fending it off, I sternly reprimanded myself that catastrophising the situation was pointless and detrimental. Wait until the words were spoken…if they were to be spoken.

Concentrating on driving was crucial, a priority, but spaces of time disappeared when my mind drifted back to appointments leading up to this moment. The concerned glance from the mammogram technician, the uncertain reassurance from the ultrasound specialist and the grave and clinical reaction from the biopsy doctor. The seemingly harmless words *'good luck'* from all of the above had taken a sinister turn. My suspicious and irrational mind added to the fear by questioning why good luck was needed.

I arrived at the breast clinic, parked and then paused to calm my thoughts. I would have given anything to stay seated in the car, protected from the future. Ignorance is bliss. Unfortunately, time didn't wait for stoic preparations, and the minutes ticking past the hour pressured me to leave my vehicular sanctuary.

The waiting room was yet another test. I picked up a magazine and blindly flicked through it without any intention of consuming its content. The waiting was long and painful, and distractions were few...

Educational campaigns on breast awareness have been advertised extensively over the past twenty years to promote the genuine need to check your breasts. As a female, it is absolutely essential, and yes, blokes can have breast cancer too, so if you are not checking, then you really should start - right now. The fact is, I didn't have a lump, or a dimple, or resemblance of orange peel, but any change in your breasts is a sign that you need to follow up with your doctor. Upon finding anything unusual, it is quite likely that you will magnify the situation, and without waiting to know the medical results, you will have a breakdown and start planning your own funeral. *'Love You 'Till the End'* by The Pogues and *'Into the Mystic'* by Van Morrison were the music for mine. Waiting on results is agonising.

It was late January 2011, a Saturday, when I woke to discover that my right nipple appeared to be bleeding. I felt totally confused as to why or how this could happen, and no matter how hard the rational portion of my brain tried to justify this bleeding, a massive alarm was loudly and persistently ringing. Shutting out this noise was almost impossible. The combination of panic, apprehension, distress and the availability to search the internet created a tsunami that unleashed and attacked my reasoning, logic, and senses. My advice is never to refer medical issues to the internet. It will offer you various scenarios that will inevitably lead you straight back into a panic, where you will convince yourself that you have the direst of diseases and death is imminent.

The weekend of assumptions finally ended, and I managed to see my GP Monday morning. No doubt she could sense my tentative approach to knowing, but avoiding a diagnosis was not an option.

There was simply no escaping. She explained that bleeding from the nipple is not a particularly common situation, but didn't appear overly concerned. The fact that the referral she wrote to the breast surgeon was marked URGENT was evidence to the contrary.

The initial breast clinic appointment with the breast surgeon was pragmatic and clinical, offering no accurate indication of any outcome, good or bad. And trust me, I was looking. Looking for anything to indicate there was a way out of this nightmare. I could have been told that bleeding from the nipple might be caused by heartburn, and I would have believed him. However, of course, the answers were never going to be determined without a multitude of tests. A mammogram, an ultrasound and then finally, a biopsy of my nipple, which by the way, was not a particularly pleasant experience. The biopsy involved being hoisted into the rafters, lying upon a table with my right breast dangling through a hole, a hole in the table designed explicitly for body parts to dangle through. The doctor then stood under the table and proceeded to insert the appropriate medical instrument into my nipple. As I said, it wasn't pleasant. Mentally speaking, well, dignity was left to cower in the corner and was forcibly replaced by detached indifference. Ultimately, my awkward horror at having to dangle my breast through a hole in a table was simply unimportant.

It then became a waiting game. The rules of this game were minimal and straightforward. I became totally possessed with unrelenting emotion and unable to focus on anything other than a foreboding outcome. The longer it takes for results to be known, the longer you are left in limbo. It is the place where your imagination takes hold, and you cannot move forward until the dice is rolled again.

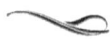

Finally, I was called to follow the breast surgeon into his room and then sat in a fog of disbelief as he explained my situation.

It was indeed breast cancer. A somewhat rare type, less than four per cent and called Paget's disease of the breast. The surgeon then drew some primitive diagrams and explained the urgent need to remove my right breast. The details of forthcoming medical procedures were unable to penetrate my brain. I was aware that this information was essential, and I should try to concentrate on his words. Instead, I simply sat there. I was hovering in a place that was somewhere between reality and delusion. My mind appeared to have wandered into another realm. A place that was separated from my body, floating somewhere nearby but not attached. For a moment, my entire existence was not present. It was replaced by an enveloping protective numbness that allowed me to retard the emotion - for now.

Whilst my intuitive voice had tried to warn me, there really was no preparation for this.

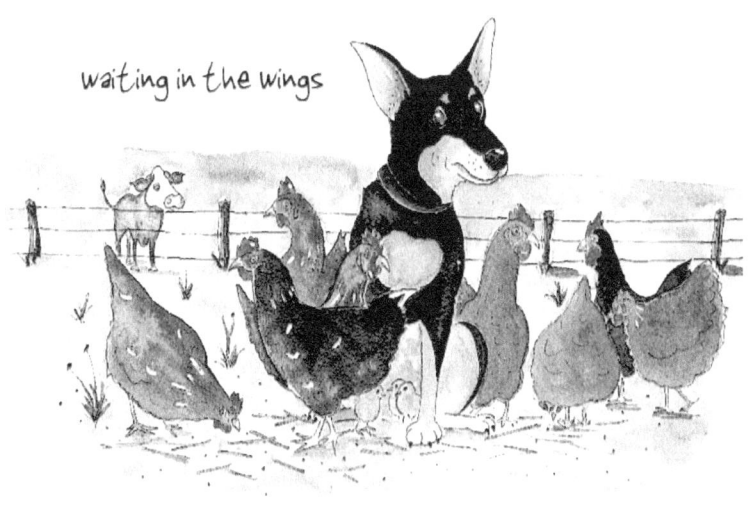

waiting in the wings

Wednesdays with Harry
IN ART WE TRUST

What does it say when your son declares that a trip to the National Gallery of Victoria is where he would like to spend today? Unless alien artistic culture gremlins infiltrated his brain during the night, the only explanation is that we are having a scheduled power cut, which, of course, would end all forms of life as he knows it.

Harry had heard that the current exhibition was worth a gander and so, with very little research, realised that it ended on Sunday and had free entry. Perhaps he should have researched a little further to discover that you still needed a ticket, and school holidays meant hordes of desperate parents seeking free holiday entertainment were also on the prowl. So now I found myself questioning whether the pull to experience another mother-son art gallery encounter was greater than the hassle of driving 1.5 hours, navigating traffic, finding parking, queuing, and crowds, all while nursing a head cold.

Side note: During a global Covid pandemic, it is not wise to acquire a cold/flu, cough, sneeze, hay fever, allergies or anything that indicates such symptoms. The consequences from the sneeze police are stares, glares, judgement, and condemnation that are undoubtedly without sympathy and more akin to punishment, such as burning at the stake. I did, in fact, had a Covid test on Monday. Yes, it was negative. Perhaps they should also issue a T-shirt announcing such results.

After queuing for a ticket and then queuing to enter, I realised that many of this art-loving population simply sought where next to queue. Was it the queue to the toilet or the queue to look at the miniature sculptures that persuaded and encouraged this pied piper approach? From desperate bladder-bursting looks, particularly from middle-aged females, I quickly surmised that those looking for the loos were horrified to find themselves herded into any lines that formed and were sadly standing in front of a tiny sculpture instead of sitting down to pee.

This latest NGV exhibition aimed to offer a unique, thought-provoking view of the world from various artists, some known, some up-and-coming, all displaying different perspectives and genres. It was a diverse collection of art, design, science, and technology seemingly wrapped up in a statement. The overwhelming theme encompassed subjects such as race, gender, environment, climate, social inequality, you know, all the big ones. There appeared to be an emphasis on pushing the traditional boundaries of what actually constitutes art, and that is why I found myself staring (although somewhat briefly) at a chair covered in blue plastic shards and indeed questioning, *'What is Art?'* Harry was standing next to me, looking at a stack of PVC pipes, and his judgement was not so philosophical. His assessment of that particular display was, *'what the fuck?'* Actually, that was his assessment for many of these exhibits.

I often find myself people watching when attending such events. It was evident that this particular crowd could be divided into three distinct groups.

First was the already recognised parents with young children, attempting to occupy another day in the holidays that was free of charge and who were desperately hoping the Wiggles were on display. They walked rapidly through the gallery sniffing out anything bright, colourful and kiddy-friendly that would appease little Mason, Harper, Logan or Amari, and they breathed a sigh of relief when discovering the vivid oceanic exhibit. Whilst its theme was regarding toxic waste in marine life, the humungous orange octopus created from hand-felted cigarette butts was a big hit with the kids. Perhaps the massive polystyrene coffee cup hovering skyward filtered in the message of waste products, or maybe it was simply a fun object gawked at by the kids before they started chanting for Maccas.

The second is the '*We are here, but not sure if enjoying it*' group. This is Harry's people. They have heard it worthwhile and so took the risk. They question why so many people were there with young kids, troubled themselves about the length of queues, open-minded enough to look at all the exhibits, yet judgemental enough to think much of it pointless. Find reading the blurbs a little too taxing, so take a random guess at the purpose and mostly declare, '*what the fuck?*' They encounter Pinocchio's Reality, a row of different-sized noses and are confused about how it relates to power, politics and perception. They walk down the dark hall to trigger the air dancer, but with all due respect to its artistic concept, they find the giant inflatable prop more associated with used car lots. They honestly don't care to watch the video of a sleepless girl in bed, wrapped in her doona, sending texts into cyberspace regarding her love life. They finally feel at home when they enter a room full of sporting trophies, only to learn their inscriptions are focused on racism and classism and clearly scoffing at the obsession with triumph and competition. They ponder over metal tapestries claiming that '*You are Not Tequila*' and they gravitate towards the interactive exhibits such as the Humming Room- an empty room with a security guard out front and simply the instruction, '*To enter the room, you must hum a tune. Any tune will do.*' If they wanted to look at fine porcelain plates, they would watch Antiques Roadshow; however, they did enjoy the shoelaces creating the '*Last Words of John Brown*'. And finally, they believe creating their own art by taking a photo of their shadow is essential to complete the visit. All in all, they are glad they went but would rather watch the footy or go to the pub.

The third group are true art lovers. They are easily recognised by their crushed linen uniform and no-care hairstyle. They are genuinely there to spend as much time as necessary to ascertain every detail and underlying nuance from every piece of work. They have their NGV membership card tattooed on their forehead and walk with a calm yet determined stride. They know exactly where to find the toilets without a queue, and they are experienced at seeking out the limited seating. They sit and contemplate the artist's views and intricacies and appear to accept that art is whatever it needs to be. The creative practice of this changing landscape reveals a new paradigm, and they are up to the challenge. They have no desire to eat at Maccas, nor do they need to photograph their shadow.

So there you go...

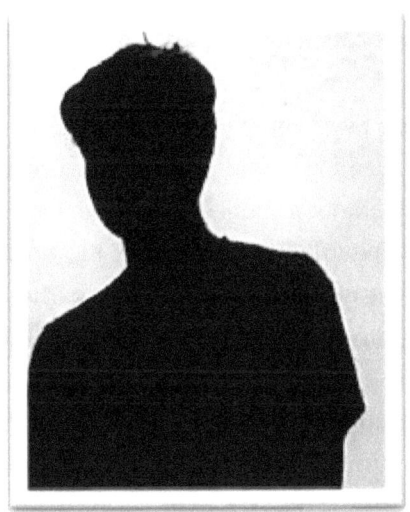

UP IN THE AIR

I was once again seated in the refuge of my car, but this time, there was little hope of calming my thoughts. I was desperately trying to cling to anything rational. I phoned Bryce (husband) at his work. The conversation was brief; talking was difficult, god, simply breathing was difficult.

The urge to immediately seek the love and support of family was strong, and the drive from the breast clinic to my parents' house was about twenty minutes. Miraculously, I steered the car without incident. It was only when the ignition was safely turned off that I allowed myself to let go. The force of emotion that rattled my being came with an impact that churned my stomach, pounded my head and was unlike anything I could remember.

My sisters were called and rushed to Mum and Dad's to surround me with support. I knew that this would affect more than just me, and as a parent myself, I was very aware of how this news would distress my own parents. Feeling helpless when the world closes in on your child is a weighty emotion and leaves you vulnerable to feelings that are beyond anything tolerable. However, their own emotions were put on the back burner in order to build a barrage of comfort.

No one was prepared for this, so all that could be done was to attempt to be as reasonable as possible and deal with what we knew, as well as the practical issues that needed to be put in place.

I was brought up in a household where pragmatism was always sought and preferred. Function over form. A reliable notion that offered stability when drama gets in the way. It becomes a lifeline to lucidity when ambiguity, confusion and chaos threaten to run amok.

It was difficult to ascertain what the future would mean because I had not clearly understood all the details. My only focus was that I had cancer and that people died from cancer. That idea simply led to the enormous, neon-flickering billboard exploding in my mind, which read, 'What about Harry?'

Harry, my only child and, at that time, eleven years old. All I could think of was him growing up without a mother, and no matter how much I tried to apply some level-headed reasoning, the dark side was closing in. The fact was, it wouldn't be until after the operation that we would know what stage the cancer would be classified, if it had spread and if it was curable.

I wish I knew then what I know now. Firstly, if you're going to die of cancer, it won't be from early detected cancer, it will be when it is advanced and incurable, and secondly, it is not over till it is over.

By the way... I do realise the word *curable* is quite a curious one in the cancer world. Some view that you are *cured* if you stick around for a predetermined number of years, and there is NED (No Evidence of Disease). Others say there isn't a cure but that you may be in remission. Of course, there is always the possibility of cancer returning, even after many years of being cancer-free. Tell me that cancer is not going to kill me, and I'm okay. Perhaps if you have an optimistic prognosis, you could at least be cured of constant fear and not hold on to dread. I tend to be quite basic when talking about cancer and speak in simple terms, such as curable or incurable. I understand it is more complex, but it does seem that we tend to plonk all prognosis or stages of cancers in the one big bucket regarding the fear that is generated.

Harry has faced his own challenges in life and has made significant progress in overcoming them. Many of the adopted theories that have helped him have also greatly benefited me. He would be an excellent mentor, inspiring others with his knowledge and tools for overcoming anxieties and stresses. I do, however, respect his thinking and believe that it is his own story to tell. Nevertheless, when I was first diagnosed, I knew that I needed to protect him from anything threatening, and right now, that meant that I had to pull myself together as it was time to pick him up from school.

The conversation was relatively short. I explained that I needed an operation and may not feel great for the next twelve months, but ultimately, I would be fine. Harry took that at face value and seemed okay. You could argue that kids are resilient and don't credit them enough for coping with such impacts. Harry wasn't like most kids, and I knew in the deepest depths of my soul that if I couldn't survive this, then he would be seriously affected and retreat to a place beyond reach.

There is no doubt in my mind that the strength and determination that was vital to find, along with the need to retain independence, was and is absolutely due to my love for Harry. Curiously, cancer provided a reason for us both to embrace resilience and taught us the importance of remaining present.

The rest of that day was somewhat cloudy. I left it to my family to contact close friends and let them know the outcome, as I could not converse without becoming upset. Tears were shed and seemed to be attached to the spoken word.

I also recall another prominent thought that lingered in my head that day: the belief that I would never laugh again.

I simply couldn't see the light.

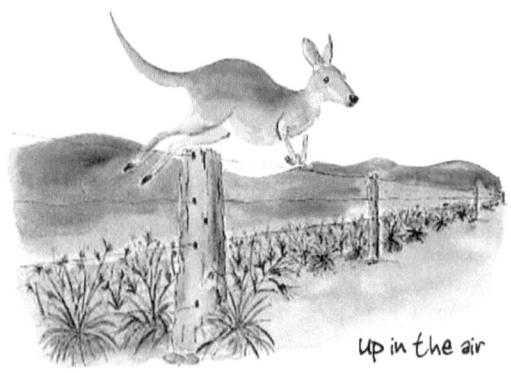

up in the air

Wednesdays with Harry
FLAT-PACK PANDEMONIUM
March 13-15,

We began the day with one simple objective in mind. Buy Harry a desk. Harry needed a desk to encourage him to stop using the coffee table as his study area.

The challenge to take on the task of a DIY flat-pack was confidently proposed by Harry, and so there was never really a question about where we would shop for this desk. Not wanting to suppress this rare and infrequent creative zest and enthusiasm, I quickly adopted a stoic attitude and off we popped into the world of multifarious mazes of household furniture and chattels that is, of course, IKEA. All you could possibly need to furnish a house, and then some, was exhibited under one roof.

Harry seemed to take delight in everything IKEA. From the 286-page catalogue to the showrooms full of household displays, the market hall exploding with domestic bliss, the plastic dispensers full of free stubby pencils, to the queue in the café to score a Kolsyrad Appeldryck and cheap lunch (no, not the meatballs). I explained very clearly that this was to be a short visit, find the desk and escape. Silly me. You enter the showroom area, and immediately, the memories of past shopping ventures tickle your subconscious. You know something is looming, and then it hits you. You have NO alternative but to spend the next hour and forty-five minutes robotically following arrows, squinting at signs, then pleading with the staff and begging strangers, JUST LET ME OUT!

If anyone is obsessed with fulfilling their daily step count, try visiting IKEA and exploring the shortcuts. There are none. Before you know it, you have spun around, increased your footprint, and are enticed to purchase bookshelves, sofa beds, dining chairs, and cooking pots.

So, after countless steps and much frustration later, we finally spied the desk section and selected an appropriate desk. THEN: - located the free pencils and noted the self-help location number; realised didn't need a pencil, could just take a photo; followed the arrows aimlessly behind a mother with two energetic kids and a young couple looking for a futon; trudged through the endless muddle of a market hall; lost Harry in the lighting section, found him patting a fluffy rug; located the flat-pack desk; loaded it on a trolley; paid at the checkout; realised the trolley with desk couldn't leave the shop area; left Harry with the desk to go find the car; drove to the loading bay but no sign of Harry; phoned Harry but he doesn't answer; cursed a few times; left the car to find Harry standing oblivious at the other end of the planet; transferred shopping from boot section to back seat; cursed again; realised desk box would not fit in unless blocked the rear-view; didn't care, just get the thing in the car!!!

One may have come to believe it was the shopping trip itself that caused angst. Not so. The fun had only just begun. I realised that Harry hadn't actually attempted to DIY flat-pack assembly until now. With the first bravado statement, *'don't need the instructions,'* still lingering in the air, Harry's love of this furniture expedition was rapidly slipping away.

The assembly took place over two days. The instructions that were arrogantly tossed aside were now relocated, perused and then repeatedly abused. Fortunately, the strength and durability of these instructions were outstanding and could be de-wrinkled and re-scrutinised.

'I HATE FLAT-PACKS' was the echoing chant as small wooden pegs, allen keys and screws were tossed about the room. The realisation that the drawers, finally assembled, were, in fact, back-to-

front, was most likely the low point. The reality of correcting such an error created a tipping point that took enormous encouragement and determination to proceed. So… after many, many hours and much suffering from all concerned, finally a desk was born.

Well done Harry, and yes, there were quite a few spare parts. So there you go...

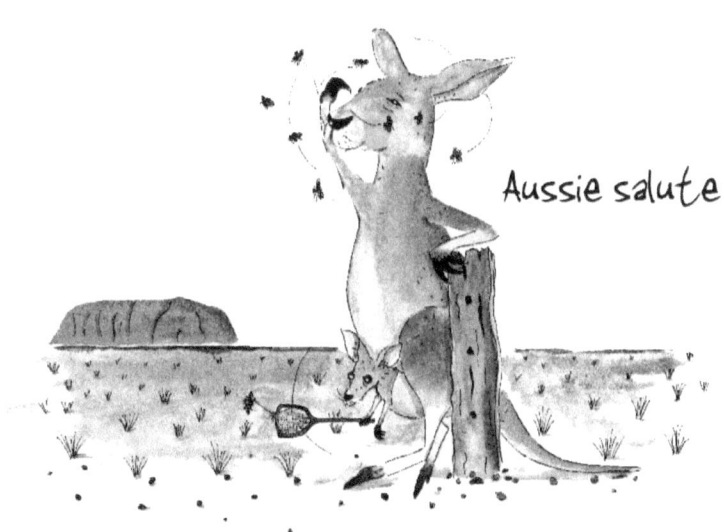

Aussie salute

OFF WITH HER BREAST!

With very little research on my behalf and complete faith in medical science, I agreed to a full mastectomy of my right breast. I was told that it was too long an operation to attempt any sort of reconstruction, which may or may not happen later. Full axillary clearance of my lymph nodes under my armpit would also be done. Therefore, the right side of my chest would be void of any resemblance of a breast, including my nipple, and it was likely that I would be permanently numb under my armpit.

Early morning, March 7th, 2011, Bryce drove me to the hospital, and the surgical preparation began.

The only other operation I had experienced before this was an emergency appendectomy at the age of twenty-one. My appendix had burst, and once it was established that it wasn't a severe indigestion crisis, I was rushed to hospital. Apparently, I was pretty lucky that the rushing took place. Still, my only recollection leading up to that surgery was the vague mention that keyhole surgery was not an option and the question, *'where does it hurt?'* - And then I blanked out.

I soon discovered on the morning of March 7th, that a planned surgery required quite a long preparation and that anything medically related entailed a great deal of waiting, hence the genuine need to title a room specifically for doing just that. I cannot tell you how many hours since, that I have spent in this room - the waiting room. I believe the term 'patient' must have derived from the amount of patience needed due to the relentless and constant waiting that patients are indeed required to do. I passed the time by people watching.

From a young age, in moments of curiosity or boredom, I have entertained myself by playing a game I call *Scrutiny*. No winners and no rules. The only fundamental objective is to notice people and attempt to imagine their lives. Sometimes I change it up a little and establish a story from simply observing their shoes. Of course, the outcome is full of assumptions and conceptions that are only true in my ideation. Now don't be alarmed; it is not at all stalky or pervy, simply fulfilling my curious and speculative mind. I still play this game to this day, and just last week, when driving, I pulled up at the traffic lights and was adjacent to a metallic blue Camry with an elderly couple. I imagined their names were Walter and Dorothy, Dot for short. They have been married for fifty-nine years and are just returning home from grocery shopping. Dot is driving because Walter has recently been suffering from a touch of gout in his knee. They are discussing the idea of having mashed pumpkin with their corned beef tonight, but they didn't buy pumpkin because neither of them had the strength to cut it up. Perhaps they should buy the already cut and prepared pumpkin next time, but that did cost quite a lot more. Mashed potatoes would have to do. And just as other vegetables were about to be debated, the lights changed, and I had to drive ahead, leaving Dot and Walter to dawdle behind. Yes, *Scrutiny* is tainted with stereotype suppositions.

I observed people coming and going into the waiting room, and let my mind wander. Which bits of their bodies were about to be explored? Was anyone else here to have cancer chopped out? I concluded that the middle-aged gentleman shifting from side to side on the chair in the corner was Mark and was here for colorectal surgery. Across from me was Charlie, a confident young woman, rapidly typing texts on her phone, impatiently waiting with her mother, Judy. Judy sighed. She was accustomed to her daughter's impatient character and wasn't surprised when she approached the nurse for the third time to insist that it was taking too long to be seen. It was Judy who needed a hysterectomy. And so it goes.

The nurses were all very friendly and offered reassuring calmness. Years of experience showed, and they instinctively seemed to know who needed the most support. Finally, they called my name, and I entered the next section, where clothes were stripped and placed in a pale blue plastic bag. In their place was an ill-fitting hospital gown requiring contortionist skills to bind the ties; paper underwear that clearly were incapable of protecting modesty; compression stockings that needed levers and pulleys to apply; and a loosely woven head net akin to working in a deli. It would actually be quite comical if I weren't being prepared for a serious operation.

Eventually, I was introduced to the orderly who would be transporting me to the operating theatre. Another kind soul who offered the necessary distracting chitchat and a comforting smile. The bed was transformed into a mobile trolley, and with the steely barriers yanked up in place, we were finally on our way. Of course, the bars were there to prevent patients from falling off; however, I did wonder if their presence also deterred and prevented potential escapees. I noticed the dull colours and chipped paint on the walls where beds have clashed and crashed along the corridors. The fluorescent lights penetrated my vision, and the chatter from above seemed distant and muffled. My mind was cluttered with questions and thoughts, but oddly not about what life would be like without a breast. It just didn't seem to have occurred to me to consider how that would feel. My only thoughts were about eradicating cancer, that fearful beast that was cunningly plotting to infiltrate my life in the most horrendous way. It simply had to be destroyed at all costs. The anaesthetist introduced herself and set about locating a suitable vein. It wasn't easy. I have crap veins. Finally, I was ready, and the countdown to oblivion began.

The following day, I was told that it was a difficult operation. At some point during that day, I think my body went into shock. For what seemed like hours, although wasn't, my body trembled and quivered in uncontrollable convulsions. My conservative approach to life dictated that I not make a fuss; however, panic and alarm overruled and pushed the alert button. A nurse swiftly attended. She checked vitals and confidently concluded that all was well. She told me that I was fine. I disagreed. Either way, the trembling eventually subsided.

Knowing, understanding, and agreeing that a body part must be removed is very different from when it has actually been removed. The fact is, whether you have large or small breasts, like or dislike them, they are a very key physical feature that announces our gender. Removing my breast was significant on so many levels. The reason that it had to be removed was significant, the impending prognosis was significant, the pain associated with the removal was significant, the loss of feeling feminine was very significant, and the insecurities and questions were significant. The fact is, many of these issues remain significant to me even after so many years. The grief is real.

I left the hospital three days later, with a drainage tube in one hand and care instructions in the other. A week later, the follow-up appointment with the breast surgeon was where I would learn the outcome of the tests from the operation.

Trepidation conquered. It turns out that the Paget's disease I have is of the type HER2+ breast cancer. It is not the worst type, but not the best. Who knew there was a best type of breast cancer and, for that matter, different types? I also learnt cancer had spread to my lymph nodes, which put me in the stage three category. Apparently, I was quite unlucky as the amount of cancer was small but unfortunately quite aggressive, and the chances of it returning were high.

Since my veins were in hiding, it was suggested that a portacath be inserted in the left side of my chest. This would then be accessed for all future treatments and scans. It required another operation. I agreed to have it done immediately before my first chemo treatment. I was also told that I needed to become steelier and that it was no point worrying about the future, and hey, none of us knows what the future brings.

I then met an Oncologist who explained my impending treatment. Six months of AC and Taxol chemotherapy, followed by seven weeks of daily radiotherapy and twelve months of Herceptin, a targeted therapy. It was also suggested that I take part in a DCare clinical trial that could help others in the future. I agreed to participate, and part of that trial allowed for yearly full-body MRI scans. The breast care nurse followed up with a myriad of brochures and pamphlets, care packages, breast prosthesis information and a hug.

The amount of information was overwhelming, but, in some way, created a welcome distraction from the very reason it was needed. I left the breast clinic that day knowing that the news could have been better, but it also could have been worse.

The real question in facing a cancer diagnosis is whether or not you have time. Time to live. I wasn't looking forward to the coming months of treatment, but I knew I would do anything to negotiate more time.

pear-shaped

Wednesdays with Harry
PANDEMICALLY SPEAKING

Okay, so the idea behind Wednesdays with Harry was that I could spend more time with my son. Little did I know that would now mean ALL the time. The COVID-19 virus appears dire, and we are all subjected to following the restrictions and advice; this is not about making light of the current circumstances. HOWEVER!

Needless to say, our usual activities will be put on hold for now as we adjust to the new normal. In their place will be me attempting to encourage Harry to partake in some board games, in-depth conversations, creative hobbies, cleaning skills and a spot of cooking. The reality will be Harry detesting board games, grunting out one-word sentences, lifting weights, going for countless runs, creating the need to clean, watching reruns of The Office, and complaining that he is hungry. His university is now online, and so the excuse for spending time in his room, in his mind, is now justified.

As I am somewhat in the crappy category for immune deficiencies, I thought it wise to take Harry grocery shopping with me as some sort of human germ shield, and yes, I do realise that is quite the oxymoron statement. He strongly objected to coming, but his need to purchase some hair goo altered his decision. Last time, I apparently bought gel instead of putty. Yes, there is a difference. He explained that whilst the outside containers looked similar, the putty was white inside. I, of course, informed Harry that it was highly unlikely that I would park my trolley in the men's toiletry section whilst I proceeded to open various hair products with the aim of detecting their colour. He begrudgingly tagged along.

So the first step in this new age of shopping is the trolley itself. I figure that the least amount of my person touching it will be beneficial, so pry one off the steely ranks with my fingertips. I then use the same fingertips, and on occasion, my elbow, to manoeuvre and steer my chariot while simultaneously being mindful of the 1.5-metre distance from fellow shoppers and not to touch my face. Of course, the fact that I shouldn't touch my face instantly creates the most annoying itch on my nose.

The first thing I spy is someone checking out with an eight-pack of toilet paper. My heart skips a beat, and I quickly change directions to seek out a couple of pallets overflowing with loo rolls that are glowing like a beacon of hope in aisle twelve. The craziness of toilet-paper-gate will perhaps never be resolved, except to conclude that the human race are idiots. So I grasp onto the one pack allowed and feel calm in the knowledge that any plans of hunting lavatory necessities could subside, at least for another two weeks.

Now my thoughts shift to what else was essential. We cruise up and down the aisles with more reassurance that the panic buying had dissipated somewhat, that is, on most items. Of course, soap is hard to find, and apparently, dry biscuits are proving popular. It says a lot when the only packets left adorning the shelves are fibre boosting rye crispbreads. Harry informed me that if ever he wanted to eat cardboard, he would chew on the box. I question my need to purchase another can of tuna and second-guess the necessity for more luxury items such as razors and lip gloss. Now I understand that staying home allows one to neglect one's upkeep, but do I really wish to surrender all maintenance? Perhaps not just yet. I imagine at the end of this, we will all exit our homes looking like we have been saved from a desert island; bearded, unkempt, dishevelled and incoherently calling for a volleyball named Wilson.

Well, we manage to navigate the aisles, untouched and unbreathed upon and go to line up on a bit of tape marked on the floor for the checkout queues. It was about this time that I realised that numerous shoppers were waiting and only two checkouts were open. Evidently, I needed to use all my experience to deduce whether queue number one, with more items in trolleys, but a quick checkout assistant, would beat queue number two, with fewer goods but a quite chatty, slow register operator. Harry was confused and strongly disagreed with my choice of queue number one. So the challenge was on, and for some time, Harry had that, *I told you so,* look on his face, and his objections were not too subtle. I held firm, and we finally managed to complete our transactions ahead of those in queue two. Victory was mine. I smugly pushed the trolley (with fingertips) back to the car, vindicated and justified.

The celebration was short-lived. Among the random collection of phone chargers, breath mints and car manuals, I searched the glove box for a packet of hand wipes. I quickly realised that the resealable opening was, in fact, not at all resealable, which, of course, meant they were entirely dried up and utterly ineffective in sanitising my hands. I needed another plan to disinfect my contaminated fingertips and finally scratch my nose. ARGH!

So there you go...

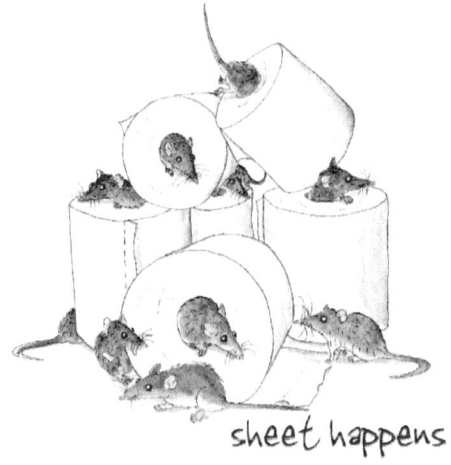

sheet happens

REACTIONS – UNDER AND OVER

How does anyone react to the news that someone they care about has been diagnosed with cancer? Initially, it didn't occur to me to ascertain that knowledge because, at the time, I was too caught up in the whole *'cancer is going to kill me'* campaign.

Looking back, I most likely overreacted to my initial diagnosis. I knew nothing about reacting to cancer except how our society often views any cancer diagnosis, and that is with terror and fear. Not that my reaction was unacceptable; in fact, it would have been considered entirely appropriate and even relatively moderate. Generally, I think we tend to react first and figure it out later. I often wonder if we reduce the fear of cancer, would the reaction lessen and vice versa. I get it, though. It is scary, and for many, a cancer diagnosis may mean insidious treatment, painful side effects and, of course, can ultimately result in death. However, I know that learning how to cope more reasonably and resolutely is so much more beneficial for my mental health. Until we all become a little more educated on cancer and change the cancer speak, there is an expectation that a cancer diagnosis will automatically receive the full deluge of grief from all involved. The patient will be horrified, and friends and family will be mortified - no matter what stage is the prognosis. Finding a middle ground is difficult.

Therefore, it came as no surprise that the outpouring from friends and family, along with genuine sympathy, shock and tearful sorrow, was the offer of help. The collection of casseroles and soups grew as we navigated our way into a new phase of a relationship.

I am blessed to have family and friends who would have no issue picking up the phone at four in the morning if it meant quelling my fears. Whilst that hasn't actually been necessary, I know if needed, it is there. And in a way, that is really all you need. A simple promise to be there.

This quote from Ernest Hemingway pretty much sums it up...
'In our darkest moments, we don't need solutions or advice. What we yearn for is simply human connection—a quiet presence, a gentle touch. These small gestures are the anchors that hold us steady when life feels like too much. Please don't try to fix me. Don't take on my pain or push away my shadows. Just sit beside me as I work through my own inner storms. Be the steady hand I can reach for as I find my way. My pain is mine to carry, my battles mine to face. But your presence reminds me I'm not alone in this vast, sometimes frightening world. It's a quiet reminder that I am worthy of love, even when I feel broken. So, in those dark hours when I lose my way, will you just be here? Not as a rescuer, but as a companion. Hold my hand until the dawn arrives, helping me remember my strength. Your silent support is the most precious gift you can give. It's a love that helps me remember who I am, even when I forget.'

So, it turns out that having cancer is the epitome of the elephant in the room. My stance has been to try to minimise any awkwardness by taking the lead. Others tend to respond to how you react and behave, and I have generally tried to alleviate that uneasiness by adopting an open-book approach. It isn't about always being solid and unflinching; it is about growing together with knowledge and awareness and, yes, sometimes fear and emotion. My team now knows that if I want to discuss cancer, I will; if not, it's business as usual.

The clue is in the title of this book, but for me, it is absolutely about chasing normal. Normality dispels and contradicts cancer's need for attention. It isn't about completing bucket lists or living each day as if it were your last; it is about the simplicity, the routines, and the normality of life. That may mean driving the Amalfi Coast or swaying to Andre Rieu performing in Maastricht will be left unfulfilled. But more importantly, washing the dishes may just save me from the dominance and power that cancer demands.

When I think back to the initial diagnosis, the response of shock and sorrow came from far and wide. Over the years, however, the impact of my having cancer has subsided and ultimately thinned out the herd. Now my network of friends has dwindled to the basic core, and it is only those closest to me who know the depths and bear the brunt. Others are still there, but some have taken a more peripheral approach, and perhaps that is just how it needs to be. Maybe it is how it would be with or without cancer. It would be impossible to function if a continuous shroud of concern and sympathy surrounded me. Compassion is always appreciated, but it comes at a price. It is usually linked to emotion, and excessive sorrow can become contagious, ultimately mentally tiring. Understanding, awareness and education, on the other hand, is always necessary. And really - if I wanted to let cancer define me, then I could, and it would.

A few friends have perhaps found the whole cancer world too confronting and have faded away completely. Ultimately everyone has their own lives to live, and whilst having cancer is a daily issue with me, it isn't something that interferes or affects others too significantly. I would be kidding myself to think that it would.

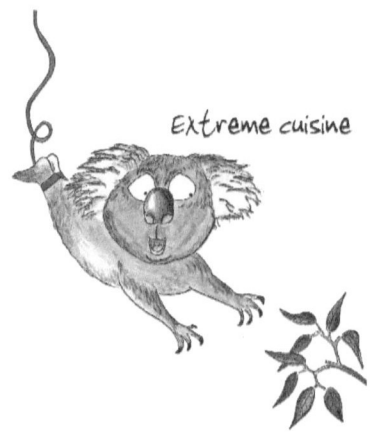
Extreme cuisine

Wednesdays with Harry
TRUE BLUE

Going to watch Carlton play AFL football is not a usual Wednesdays activity as it is an outing that we share regularly and, of course, is not on a Wednesday. Anyway, on Saturday, we ventured to Geelong for the last match of the season. Best of luck to anyone supporting the eight teams remaining in the finals. Well, that is actually not entirely sincere for Richmond, Collingwood, and Essendon. It is a compulsory contractual clause for Carlton supporters to refrain from encouraging further success for these teams. Firstly, we could be overtaken with premiership wins, and secondly, we are intense rivals and cannot feel anything but derision and contempt.

Geelong - the second largest Victorian city and seventy-four km from Melbourne. Its football team seems to think this distance is insurmountable to play where everyone else does, and so has developed their own football sanctuary where only Geelong players and supporters are allowed to penetrate. They recently redeveloped their stadium and updated the grandstands, but it seemed they overlooked the benefits of car parking and shelter.

The day began with Harry playing his own last football match for the season. The time between the end of his match and the start of Carlton playing Geelong was limited, so for Harry it was a rapid change in the car and a necessary spray of deodorant as we sprinted down the M1.

It was always going to be a challenge to find a car park. Along with hundreds of other hopeful car-parkers, we unsuccessfully cruised the backstreets, me cursing at the overwhelming build-up of traffic and Harry cursing at everyone living in Geelong. The stress was rising as game time was fast approaching. Thankfully, I managed to turn a corner, and the Boy Scouts were offering a park in exchange for $10. Bargain! So we bolted from the car, had the presence of mind to grab a couple of raincoats and joined the myriad of Geelong supporters in a queue to enter their arena.

It's quite an experience watching football at Geelong. The hordes of supporters are, of course, predominantly Geelong followers. They only seem to allow a token couple of hundred opposition supporters in the stadium, and at this point, I was yet to determine if we were privileged or not to be two of them. This question was quickly answered as we spotted the small enclosure out in the open, which was Carlton's allotment, and we totally understood where we ranked. So, we made our way to the second row of seats, one and two, that nudged up against the player's race. We were right in the action, but soon discovered we were also right among the most annoying array of football supporters.

Now, don't get me wrong, I am exceptionally well-experienced and understanding of the various types of football fans. Except when I was travelling, I cannot think of a period in my life that I haven't attended full seasons of football and, of course, witnessed every display of noise and emotion possible. From thunderous, righteous parents hanging over the fence to scream at little Nathan's suburban match, to standing in the outer at Princes Park next to a bloke who was attempting to pee in a tinny. From hearing umpires and players being harassed and abused, to children howling over one-point losses (actually, that is not just reserved for kids). The disinterested girlfriend chatting on her phone, to the grandma who has the skill to watch, yell, and crochet in unison, and the teen selling hot pies to gain access to the ground. Hell, I can even remember the days when cans were collected for cash and the cry of *'Perna, peanuts...twenty cents a bag'* from the Peanut Man echoed around the ground. The sights, the smells, the noise, the peanut shells, the emotions - I am oh so familiar with them, and they are absolutely a part of our game. So when I say they were the most annoying array, it is perhaps more a collection of the norm.

The groups of supporters at this match were divided in their actions, yet united in their annoying effect. Seated in the front row were the groupies. Before the match, they congregated as close as possible to the player entrance in an attempt to attract the attention of players and any official-looking personnel. They proceeded to utter their guidance and counsel with the absolute understanding that their advice would be taken on board. Then, when finally seated, they seemed to believe their constant banshee-like shrieking was required or necessary for the game to continue. Additionally, there were three out-of-control, seven- to ten-year-olds seated behind us. Their high-pitched, non-stop yelling, combined with the constant kicking of our seats and hitting the metal sign reverberating beside them, was excruciating. The final straw was when they leapt up and managed to distribute potato chips in my hair. Their father appeared oblivious. The older 'wiser' supporters added to the noise by commentating, discussing and complaining about every umpire decision, and finally, we have the angry vocal twenty-year-olds who, at five-minute intervals, uniformly synchronised the word *'deliberate'*.

So when the rain came pelting down, I was hopeful that all who surrounded us would run for cover. Silly me for thinking these diehard supporters would leave. All that eventuated was that we entered a new level of a nightmare - sitting in a puddle, rain soaking through coats that were incapable of holding back the tide, and surrounded by saturated, noisy nuff-nuffs. Add to this the fact that Carlton was getting thrashed, so I felt pretty justified in suggesting we leave early. Harry would have none of it as it was Dale 'Daisy' Thomas's last match, and we were in prime position to see him be chaired off at the end. Yay.

Well, eventually, the game ended; we paid our respects to Daisy, dripped our way back to the car and spent the next hour stuck in traffic surrounding the ground.

Do we wish to go back to Geelong? Not so much.

So there you go...

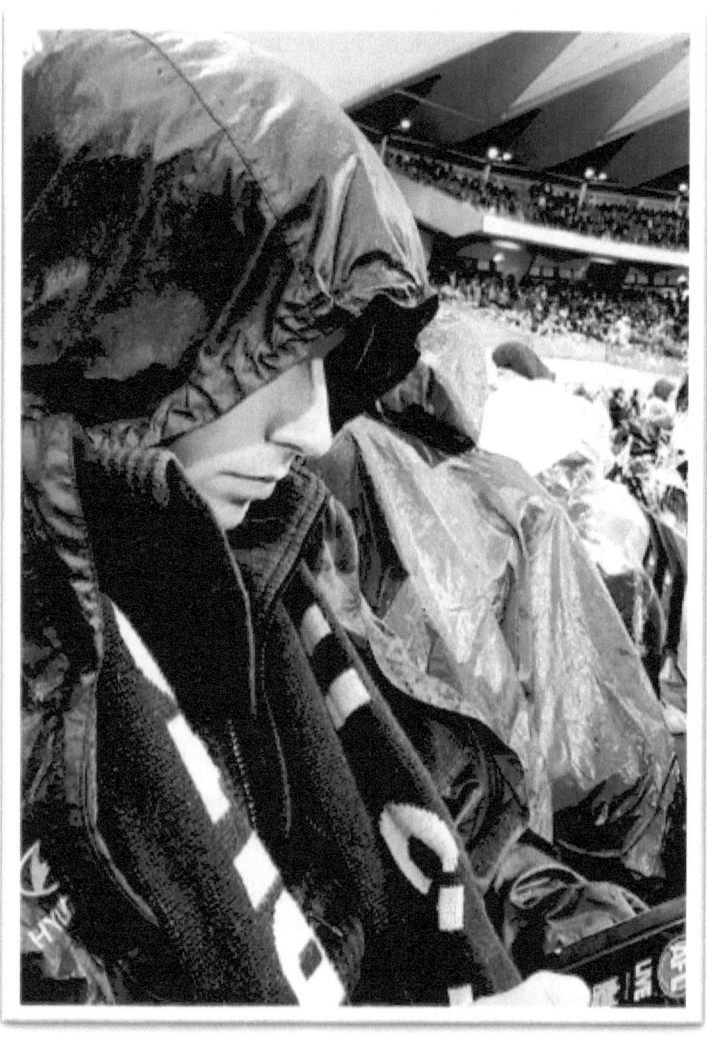

CHEMO EXTREMO

It was only a few weeks since having the mastectomy, so I was still becoming accustomed to having just one breast. I had intended to wear the large, gel-like prosthesis that I was allocated. It was held in place by being tucked in a special pocket-type arrangement within a mastectomy bra. It had been measured and supposedly weighted to match my remaining breast. I used it twice. It just didn't feel comfortable. Perhaps because it was pretty heavy and shaped like an actual breast. This meant it was in complete contradiction to my saggy southbound remaining breast and resulted in a very noticeable lopsidedness. I felt it was more evident than wearing nothing at all. So, ever since, I have elected to leave the right side of my chest void of pretend boob along with the assumption that I am of an age that my breasts, along with most other parts of my body, are pretty much inconsequential and go unnoticed. In retrospect, I think it may have been easier to have no breasts than to leave me with just one.

Chemotherapy began. The day started early as the minor operation to insert a portacath in the left side of my chest took place prior. Essentially, a vein would then be accessed via the port and alleviate the need to hunt for the more elusive veins in my arm. It has proved to be a bit of a tricky port and has had many nurses hide and take cover over the years.

With anaesthetic still fuzzing my head, I was wheeled into oncology and attempted to listen intently to the chemo briefing. The information was detailed and delivered by a beautiful nurse who had clearly presented this spiel on many occasions. She knew this overwhelming experience needed to be handled with care. So I learnt of the side effects. Some were expected to take place, and others were less likely. None were very friendly. Of course, everyone is familiar with hair loss. That doesn't always happen, but it was more likely than not with the breast cancer chemo cocktail I was on. I could expect my hair to start falling out within the first or second treatment. It was suggested that if I wanted a wig, I should sort that as soon as possible. The other cautions involved peripheral neuropathy, infections, fevers, nausea, immune deficiencies, fragile nails, teeth issues, bleeding, bruising, and the need to use steroids with their own side effects. Trying to find one positive, I did hope that surely having cancer meant that a few kilos might disappear. Unfortunately, steroids poo-pooed that idea. The anti-sickness drugs had their own set of side effects, including constipation, headaches, diarrhoea, insomnia, and indigestion. Then there was the possibility of changes to your sense of taste, smell, AND early menopause. Are you kidding me?

The last side effect mentioned was chemo brain, a genuine struggle with memory loss and focus. I managed to experience pregnancy brain, and so figured that it was similar. Well, it is, except exaggerated. I realise as we age, it may be a reasonable expectation to lose a few nouns into vocabulary's black hole, but chemo brain seems to accelerate this process. It is incredibly frustrating when you look at your garden and cannot find the actual word to describe such a plot of lawn and shrubbery without even a hint of recognition.

None of this information was meant to scare you, but you really did have to be prepared.

Well, it is safe to say that I experienced all of the above and just for good measure, menopause kicked in immediately after my first treatment. There is the theory that having side effects indicates that the chemo is doing its job. Excellent.

I realise, as I write this, that it may not appear that I am a fan of chemotherapy. I suppose it doesn't make sense to me that your immune system is torn apart and then expected to regroup and help out in the long term. It may not be in my lifetime, but I long for the day when treatment is not so destructive. I have now allowed my body to be overwhelmed by chemo twice; ultimately, it is my choice.

During this time, I felt it essential that I retain my independence as much as possible. I realise this encroached on my family's idea regarding their need to help. Sensitivities were put aside, and an understanding of how I wanted to proceed was eventually accepted. It was a natural reaction for those close by to try to alleviate stress, and at that time, they didn't feel their offerings of shepherd's pie and jelly slice were enough. They simply couldn't solve this problem and take cancer away.

I have quite a determined personality, so it shouldn't have been a great surprise that I had to do it my way. Intrinsically, I knew that I wouldn't gain the strength I felt I needed if I became too reliant and needy. Of course, there were many times I did use their help, especially on days when illness became overwhelming both physically and mentally. To me, though, it was pretty straightforward. My fortitude had to be greater than the influence cancer was asserting. That simply couldn't happen if I felt sorry for myself or spent too many days defined by cancer. The world of cancer is merely a place I am forced to visit, but it isn't where I choose to reside.

We soon all adapted to a routine. I would drive myself to chemo, and sometimes family members would come and visit, always armed with magazines and a Cherry Ripe. The car parking at the hospital was limited, so two-hour street parking was often the only option. The time they spent visiting oncology was frequently interrupted by the need to scurry about moving my car. Chemo took about five hours, depending on blood test results and waiting to see the Oncologist. I knew that I had about two hours after treatment before throwing up, so, fortunately, I was able to pick Harry up from school on my way home with enough time to spare. Harry's school was fantastic, and they accepted that I might collect him at any time.

I wasn't surprised at the consequences these chemicals had on my body. All of them had been predicted, and the side effects were living up to their promise. However, I didn't expect that the toxins would create such a disability in mobility. It was only temporary, but it was pretty difficult to walk during the last month of chemo.

The period in between treatments also fell into a pattern. The first ten to twelve days were really pretty crap, which left about a week to feel okay before the subsequent treatment sent me back to square one. There were times of stress, both physically and mentally. Hospital visits were needed when temperatures rose, and family members were called to help with anguish. So, chemo is not fun. No new information there. Again, I pray that the day comes when it is no longer needed to be the go-to treatment.

It may sound like the control freak in me completely dominated this period, but really, not so. I did learn to relax and take time for myself. We rehomed the toy trucks so my father could convert Harry's old sandpit into a meditative area. He also updated our bathroom, which allowed soothing baths to be enjoyed without peeling tiles pelting me on the head. Others helped research complimentary type therapies, including lifestyle and dietary changes. The idea that this is a time to get through and not follow a healthy diet seemed counterproductive. Now, finding that balance has come with some experimental therapies. In moments of complete desperation, I have attempted various anti-cancer regimes. The Budwig diet was a doozy! That involved eliminating almost every food substance known to mankind and replacing it with flaxseed oil and cottage cheese. I am sure I used to oil my hockey stick with what I was now required to digest, and so you will understand that after a couple of weeks, I decided food was actually needed for my existence and instead used the oil to polish my table. I am not saying any of these diets haven't helped, but I think you need to find what works for you.

There are many mixed messages regarding cancer and diets, and it bemuses me somewhat when *pinkified* products are marketed and associated with unhealthy foods or celebrations. Education on diet and mental health should go hand in hand, especially if you are in cancer treatment. It's easy to promote the idea that 'we're not here for a long time, so eat the cake and drink the wine.' From where I sit, that makes little sense. Personally, I think it's a no-brainer to strive for a healthy mind and body. I feel I am closest to actually fighting this disease when I refuse Cherry Ripes, try to eat nutritionally and practice good mental health.

So the merry-go-round of chemo continued for six months and then a further twelve months of targeted treatment. I coped. I managed to participate in regular life activities, take care of my health as much as I could, and strived for a life away from the world of cancer. Family and friends supported me, and it was and still is, so very much appreciated.

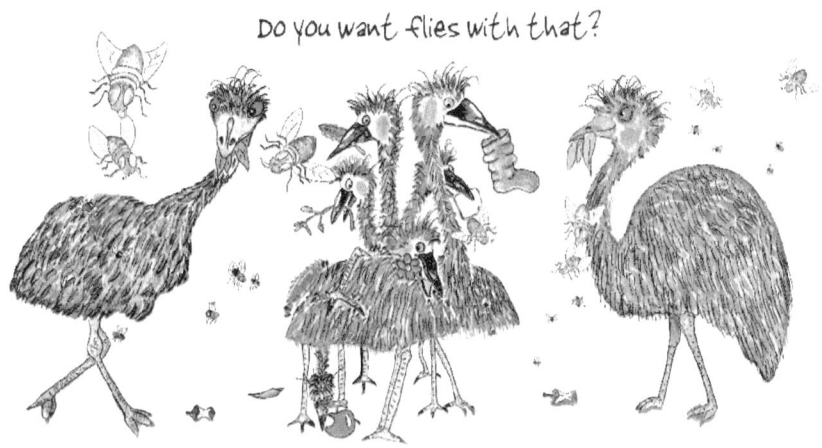

Do you want flies with that?

Wednesdays with Harry

Dear Mum

Mother's Day has come and gone, and whilst the windows didn't receive a scrub as per my usual fanciful request, I did receive a pair of slippers. Keeping my expectations relatively low is quite a handy strategy, but I did suggest Harry sort out some breakfast. Eggs and bacon were retrieved from the fridge. Then, with a degree of difficulty of an eight, he managed to flip and spin a butter-covered spatula and land it squarely on top of my fluffy right foot within five minutes of their initial foot-covered outing. Of course, it followed that Mulligan's attention was intently focused on said right fluffy slipper until all traces of food substances were licked off. You may argue that the positives are that Harry was willing to cook me breakfast and my slipper is now clean; however, the reality was that I was the one who actually finished cooking breaky, and now my new fluffy slipper was covered in dog slobber!

My gift to my mother was the latest book from ***Love Your Sister*** organisation called ***Dear Mum***. It is a collection of letters written by celebrities to their mothers, with the proceeds from sales going to cancer research. I decided to buy the book and add my own letter as a tribute.

Dear Mum,

'I have been staring at my computer for some time now, waiting for words to miraculously leap onto the screen and begin this letter to you. Only the most loving words, however, as you deserve nothing less. But where to start?

My focus is momentarily distracted by noticing the bounty of crumbs and dust that have become encrusted on the keyboard. After giving it a robust blow and then tapping it upside down, I conclude that I need to perform a more thorough cleaning method. What would you do? Well, you would most likely have specialised sprays, blowers and brushes along with a chiselling tool, sitting neatly in the adjacent drawer in anticipation of such a task. It would also occur to you to first turn off your computer. Actually, I doubt your keyboard would have the chance to collect dust, as it, along with shelves, knick-knacks, furniture and the top of the fridge, would be included in your weekly dusting routine. You have always accepted housework as a necessary duty, and we grew up not knowing any different. Fortunately, you have two other daughters who pay more attention to dusting than me!

My thoughts have now drifted into comparing our similarities. Over the years, I have been teased,

'Argh! You are just like your mother.'

Why was this meant as a criticism? If referring to your love for your family, your strong work ethics, your organisational skills, your attention to detail, your commitment to effort, your ability to cook for the masses, your generosity with your time, your craft skills, your thoughtfulness, your community contributions, your high moral standards, then YAHOO. Good on me! I dare say, though, this particular comparison was more about your stubborn tendencies and your use of THE GLARE. You have one almighty glare that can be more effective than any words spoken. My version of THE GLARE is also highly efficient and has been known to part the seas.

Your energy and accomplishments have always amazed me, and I can only hope to live up to some of your remarkable traits.

Speaking of comparisons, there are, of course, various differences in our approach to life: Your ability to organise a Tupperware cupboard is indeed masterful - I use the 'shut the door quickly before it all falls out' method. You find the time and inclination to iron tea towels - I question where my iron is. You spend hours pottering in the garden, lovingly nurturing nature - I planted hydrangeas in full sun. Your sewing ability is impressive, and you accurately follow patterns. I sew square-sleeved tops and elastic-waisted clown pants. You make an effort to be punctual - my only form of exercise is to run late. Your contribution to school fetes provided endless trays of ice-cream cone marshmallows, toffee apples and honeycomb - I organised the wine. You see dark clouds and race to rescue the washing - I see visions of elephants and Elvis. You never swear; instead, you curse with *'sugar'* and *'blast'* - I say *'shit'*. Your always 'be prepared' pantry is brimming with 'just in case someone pops in' cakes and bickies - I scrape mould off the cheese.

You are the epitome of what it means to be a mum. When needed, it is never in doubt that you are there, encouraging success, supporting and helping, fostering and inspiring, and always with an egg and bacon pie and jelly slice in hand. There has never been a time that I couldn't rely on you being there for me, and in more recent years, the challenges have been huge. You put aside your own emotions to build a strong and stable wall of reassurance.

We may not be a family that openly declares love and affection, but actions speak volumes.

Love you always Mum, **Jo** xxx

P.S...My keyboard still needs a clean!'
So there you go...

HAIR TODAY, GONE TOMORROW

I have never felt particularly confident. Growing up with rampantly thick auburn hair, a sprinkling of freckles, and a slight gap between my front teeth most likely didn't help. Sure, my Nana loved my hair and called me Stargirl, but I was the 'carrot top' or 'ranga' in the family growing up. Don't get me wrong, I didn't feel marginalised or tormented at all; in fact, I probably quite enjoyed the idea that I was a bit different and unique, and I suspect it would not surprise you to know that Pippi Longstocking was one of my favourite reads.

According to the internet, redheads make up less than two per cent of the world population, with Scotland claiming the majority. In the Middle Ages, redheaded women were thought to be witches and were burned at the stake, and the ancient Greeks believed that redheads turned into vampires after they died. Gingernut, Mark Twain once said, '*While the rest of the species is descended from apes, redheads are descended from cats.*' It is thought that redheads have a higher pain threshold than average, and research has shown that redheaded women have more sex than blondes or brunettes…finally, a benefit. Sorry ranga fellas, you not so much.   Gingerphobia is apparently an actual fear; fortunately, in more recent years, it seems the phobia has dissipated somewhat, and the appeal of having red hair has grown globally. Acceptance has flourished, and various celebrations, including National Redhead Day, Ginger Pride, and the Night of the Walking Red, are a long way from the days of stake burning. Non rangas now choose to become a redhead, and I cannot tell you how many times over the years I have been asked what colour hair dye I use.

While backpacking around Turkey in the 1980s, I became aware that my hair seemed to attract quite a lot of interest. I may have been a tad paranoid from the lingering remnants *'Midnight Express'* left polluting the air; however, I did become aware that the attention gained was in direct proportion to whether or not I wore a hat. I also know that red hair dye was used extensively by women in Moscow in late 1987. At the time, I was working for Contiki Tours and had an eye-opening experience witnessing life behind the Iron Curtain. The deprivation and scarcity of essential goods was confronting. I was in charge of food rations, and so armed with plenty of Rubles and humble curiosity, I spent many hours searching through nameless basement shops, hoping to stumble across cheese and eggs. Locals would queue for hours for whatever so-called luxury item had been recently unloaded; from toilet paper to sardines to stockings and hair dye. Actually, come to think of it, this is not a great example of women preferring to become a redhead, as I suspect their hair would be tinted blue if the latest shipment dictated.

Anyway, the crux of all this is that from early adulthood, I actually *liked* the colour of my hair. Its wiry thickness and tendency to form a curly mess was clearly not great; however, I had learned to train and tame it and had come to rely on its frizz ability to predict the forecast of rain. It had finally become one of the physical features that I felt actually looked okay.

The list of side effects from chemotherapy is long, and you must be informed thoroughly. I was told that the type of chemo I was on would most certainly cause me to lose my hair, which would happen fairly soon after treatment started. After the second round, falling strands began to weave a carpet that blanketed the bathroom floor. I remember it was actually painful to put my head on my pillow. It was like sleeping on needles. At that point, I had little choice but to face the fact that my hair wouldn't last much longer. A hairdresser friend helped out by giving me a shorter style, but it was only a week later that I had to remove the remaining locks.

I stood in the bathroom, staring at my reflection, towel wrapped tightly around my shoulders, and the Remington Power Clippers charged and ready to assault. I knew that procrastinating wouldn't change the outcome, yet I did pause for a moment. The significance of that moment suddenly became overwhelming, and I needed a moment to let it sink in. I was very aware that vanity was creeping into this emotion. I realise that many women embrace being bald and wear it like a badge of honour, and let's face it, compared to a cancer diagnosis, it is a pretty minor outcome. However, I wanted to cling to what I felt identified as me with every fibre of my being. Baldness is one of the many faces of cancer, and I simply didn't want to be branded with a look that represented it. Being treated for cancer and being ill from that treatment was onerous enough, but actually *looking* like cancer was incredibly confronting. I tried my hardest to remind myself that being bald was temporary and if being bald was what it took to combat cancer, then grieving was pointless. Had I known then that this wouldn't be the only time I had to shave my head and that today I live with hair toppers and bald patches, then I may have allowed myself to be a tad more dramatic.

Ultimately, when there is nothing you can do about a situation, the sooner you accept it, the quicker you can find peace. I finally took hold of the clippers and silently surrendered to reality. It didn't take long. I stood there with clumps of auburn locks scattered at my feet and a stranger staring back at me.

Breastless, instantly menopausal and now hairless. The challenge to feel feminine was growing. The only bonus of losing hair that I could deduce was that it meant I would be incapable of growing a beard anytime soon!

Prior to the great shave, I organised to be fitted with a wig as I figured any type of hair was better than none. I discovered that it is not until you lose your hair that you uncover the shape and size of your head. Unfortunately, no offence, Dad, but it appears that I take after my father in this department. Now, don't get me wrong with all this bald talk; many women adapt to a hairless noggin and look fantastic. I would argue, however, that they are blessed to have perfectly formed, small, round heads. My noodle does not fit into this category, as I soon discovered in trying to find solutions to head coverings. The wig that I had so carefully selected didn't seem to stay on without copious amounts of glue, specifically for wig adhering situations. The warm and steamy weather ensured that the glue struggled to cope with the furnace-like conditions cooking on my head. The final straw was when a low-lying tree branch snagged it right off my head, catapulting it skyward until it gracefully floated down and landed in a tangled mess. I took this as a sign and, at this point, put my vanity aside and began to look for alternatives. Pretty soon, the troops rallied. Beanies were knitted, scarves were gifted, and reassurances were offered with unfaltering enthusiasm.

A few months into treatment, I was invited to a morning of pampering from a wonderful organisation that understands the challenges females face when undergoing cancer treatment. Various companies donated cosmetics, and a group of female cancer patients gratefully accepted being groomed. One by one, those without hair removed their wigs, hats, and scarves, along with any cautious inhibitions. No words were needed to understand the quiet bond that was so very relevant at that moment. It was a safe space to experiment with makeup and styling headwear, guided by professionals. However, I am not sure the organisers were prepared for my peculiarly shaped noggin and most likely quickly regretted using me as their model to showcase and instruct others on headwear. Whilst there were many wigs and hats in their arsenal, nothing seemed to fit, so it soon became apparent that the lesson then shifted to what NOT to wear. The parameter of a scarf is without a definitive size, and so, with a quiet prayer to the milliner gods, they gave it a whirl and proceeded to wrap, tuck, and fold in a hundred and one ways to apply a scarf. Unfortunately, no matter what style they attempted, it simply exaggerated the irregular shape of my head. Before I knew it, I looked like a Babushka doll or a mourning widow of Latin descent. Credit due, they tried hard, but no one was convinced that my head was suited to anything other than the particular hat that I had arrived in. I had already discovered that brimmed hats with a concertina-like arrangement created the illusion of shape and a style that suited me. So, while I didn't gain in the apparel department, I really appreciated the event and the generous gesture.

In retrospect, I probably should have persisted with various wigs, as when I went through chemo the second time, I did manage to find a great line of wigs that matched my colour and length, and they fitted and stayed in place just fine.

My perspective on wearing head coverings has evolved since those early days. Looking '*normal*' is one of my key defences against the power of cancer.

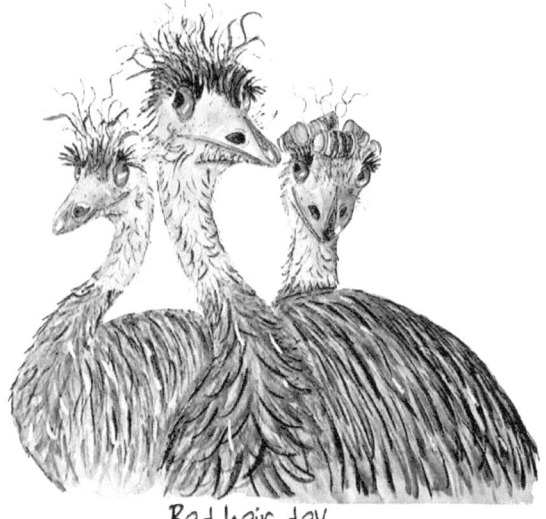

Bad hair day

Wednesdays with Harry
WHISTLER'S MOTHER

This current period of pandemic isolation and restrictions hasn't altered my day significantly. Perhaps I am one of the lucky ones, as my usual routine involves working from home. I still manage to drag myself to my office, wearing whatever attire is slung over the back of a chair, sit and munch on muesli while catching up on the latest news from my computer, and then contemplate my next project.

The Covid ramifications leave in its wake cautious health measures and a complete lack of income; however, on the whole, I am still busy preparing for life on the other side of this pandemic. The exception appears to be an overwhelming desire to bake. This, of course, is entirely at the mercy of the flour provisions available. For others in this household, the living in limbo scenario is starting to take its toll, evident from the numerous times the fridge is opened during the course of a day. The fact that our fridge has the most annoying and relentless beep when left ajar for an undetermined period of time adds to this awareness, and indeed, the predicted vocal cry *'there's nothing to eat,'* will follow.

This challenging time will be a chapter in history that we are all involved in, and the positive is that it has encouraged many to slow down and explore their creativity. The fact that jigsaw puzzles have appropriated dining room tables across the planet is a testament to this time. Not to be left out of this trend, I dusted off a cryptic one that had been languishing with other unused games and proceeded to sort the pieces. This hurdle is the first test to determine whether someone is puzzle-worthy or not. It requires a significant amount of space, patience, and perseverance—and that is just from flipping the pieces the right way up. The next step that wise puzzle gurus know is to complete the border. Now, this is when you are seduced into the mistaken belief that you will actually finish this project, as the joy of slotting pieces together is achieved with relative ease. Then, for the next six months, you will spend day after day squinting desperately in search of that elusive piece that will enable you to finish just one corner. You will convince yourself it is possible to cram the piece with three holes into the slot for two. You will question your choice of selecting such a cryptic puzzle that didn't actually show the outcome. You sneer at those passing by who declare how easy this must be, and finally, you wonder why you began it at all and then go bake a cake.

So, leaving the mystery and misery of the jigsaw puzzle aside, I wish to acknowledge all the amazing creative people this week. As a tribute to the latest art trend of sharing photos of recreations of famous paintings, I decided we would also contribute, if only in our own little world. Now, when I say we, of course, I mean Harry. I discussed the concept with him, and much like all other times he has been exposed to art, he was less than enthusiastic. I could sense that some intense negotiation would be needed for him to become involved.

After a relatively flexible agreement was in place, I then presented him with the various options. Experience and natural cunning led me to initially show him paintings that I knew he would absolutely reject. Then, I swooped in with the less offensive ones, and just like that, he agreed. So the Little Boy in Blue, Mona Lisa, The Birth of Venus and The Girl with the Pearl Earring were vehemently snubbed, leaving The Scream and Whistler's Mother to shine through. Harry did suggest that Edvard Munch would have painted The Scream after listening to his mother's crazy notions.

Cupboards were raided to create such a costume. The black attire was easy enough; however, procuring lacy headwear and cuffs proved a challenge. Finally, I discovered a stash of delicate doilies inherited from my Nana, and voila! Whistler's Mother was born.

You may notice that our version is a little taller than the original and neglected to put on shoes. Well done H!

So there you go…

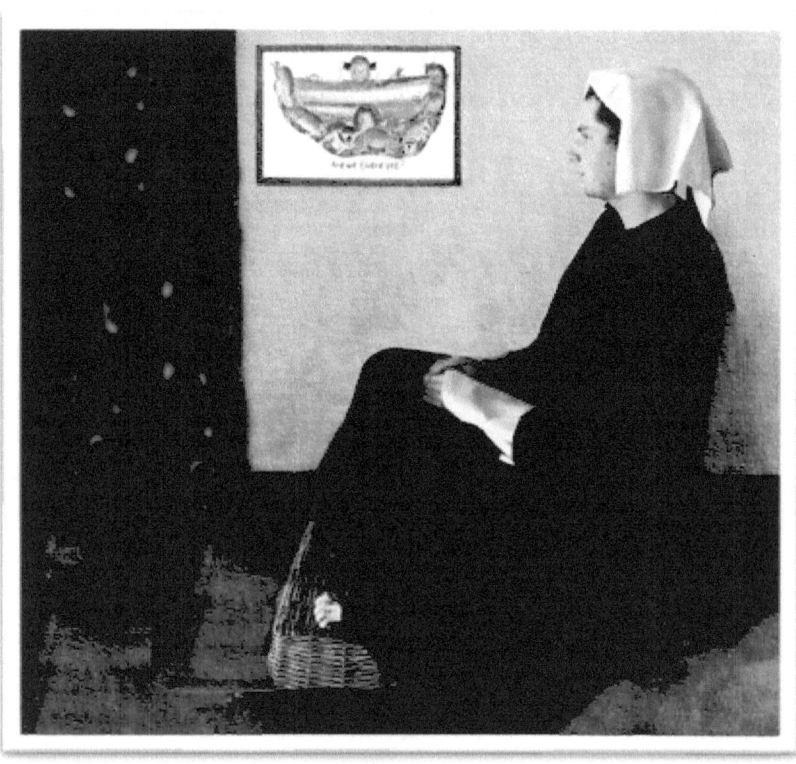

HYPNOSIS

I have always been aware that my sense of smell was above average. I can detect odours at twenty paces and can pinpoint their origin. Great to have me close by if a fire is threatening; however, not so great if you blame the dog for farting.

During the first months of chemotherapy, I agreed to partake in a study on the effect of chemotherapy on smell and taste. A side effect of chemotherapy can be the development of a lingering metallic taste. It dulls the joy of flavour, only to be replaced with the tang akin to licking a doorknob. I had learned that eating Fruit Tingles was one method to combat this tinny taste, and thanks to my sister, I was armed with a year's supply of this particular confection, which saved me from metal mouth during treatment.

This study involved smelling and tasting different vials containing various degrees of taste sensations. My task was to identify and rate the strength of taste with descriptions such as sweet, savoury, bitter, and salty. My sense of smell came along for the ride and together, with all the attributes of a bloodhound, rated off the chart. It was established that my sense of smell was in the top ninety-nine percentile and that I was a smell freak who would indeed be suffering from metal mouth.

My portacath, used as access for my chemo treatment, is located high on the left side of my chest. This means that the alcohol swab used to clean the area in preparation for the intravenous line is quite close to my face, making the smell unavoidable. It wasn't a pleasant smell, but more than that, I believe my brain began to associate that smell with chemo and mimicked the nausea sensation. Before treatment, it is necessary to undergo blood tests and have them analysed to determine if your body can tolerate the toxins that are about to be introduced. On one such occasion, my portacath was accessed, bloods taken, and it was determined that my blood count was not high enough to proceed. Now here is the fascinating bit. Usually, after chemo, I knew I had about two hours before nausea began. This time, I was driving home and had to pull over with the genuine need to throw up, yet I hadn't actually had chemo. Feeling quite chuffed that I had made an enormous discovery into some mind over matter theorem, I began to sit up and take notice. How much was a physical reaction created from my mental obstinacy and association?

I detest pumpkin, and to this day, I recall when I was eight years old and my father's warning, 'You are not leaving this table until you have eaten your plate clean,' was engraved with stern reality on a banner that hung above the table. The knowledge that I intensely disliked certain vegetables didn't seem to alter this ethos. Therefore, I sat staring at a pile of pumpkin mash for over an hour, desperately wanting to join my sisters and watch The Brady Bunch, yet unable to consume this stinky pumpkin mess. Seemingly left with no choice, I surrendered; I gripped my nose with one hand and shovelled the mash in my mouth with the other. It was less than a minute before my attempt to swallow turned into a regurgitation of bright orange proportions. After that, the banner was forever altered to allow pumpkin as a concession, followed by brussels sprouts and cauliflower.

This is not a particularly interesting story, as I am sure many kids have detested and physically reacted to certain foods. The interesting bit is that we were required to make carrot vichyssoise, a carrot soup, in high school Home Economics class many years later. I don't have an issue eating carrots; however, I simply couldn't eat it because it looked exactly like pumpkin soup. My brain knew it was made with carrots however didn't allow my swallowing devices to work. Now the question was, how could I use this metaphysical principle to my advantage? My answer was hypnosis.

I was absolutely certain that the only way I could cease feeling nauseated due to the smell of the swab was to alter my mindset somehow, and it made perfect sense to me that hypnosis could work. Before attempting such mind-altering theories, however, you would think I would have had the presence of mind to ask if a less stinky swab was available. Tripping over the obvious is indeed an issue. Anyway, I located a hypnotherapist who was also qualified in psychology, and with nonsensical notions that I would cluck like a chicken every time a dog barked, I put that to the back of my mind and proceeded with this plan.

I quickly ascertained that a swinging pocket watch wasn't an actual method to lure me into submission. Unfortunately, though, I was unable to be hypnotised for the first and remaining five sessions. To be honest, it didn't surprise me as I am quite an attentive and focused type who doesn't give up control too easily. I was simply spoken to in a very soothing and tranquil manner. There was a lot of deep breathing, and I was asked to imagine walking along a corridor…or was that a beach? Either way, the attempt to enter a deep state of relaxation was unfortunately met with resistance on my behalf. The hypnosis was then put aside, leaving my unprotected feelings and emotions to emerge.

It was far from a complete waste of time. Whilst I didn't cure my sense of stinky swab smell, it was beneficial on a deeper level. It was the first time I had spoken to a professional about how I felt about having cancer. It invited freedom of feelings. Feelings that were often stifled or restrained. Emotions were summoned and surfaced with ease. The need to protect, the need to be strong, the need to be thoughtful, and the need for resilience were not required. All that was needed was for me to release.

So with plenty of tissues on hand, a barrage of grief and sorrow escaped. It became evident that I needed to continue and embrace an emotional journey. I continue to know this and utilise mind liberation today.

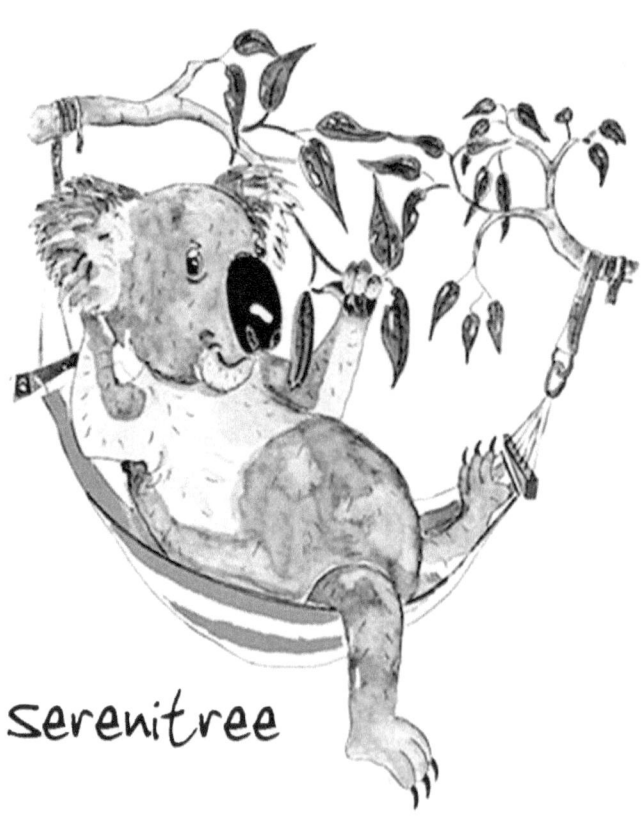

serenitree

Wednesdays with Harry
WARREN BROWN

For the past few weeks, I have fought hard to save the life of my desktop computer, Lola. She has worked tirelessly over the past ten years, rarely complaining about the incessant work overload, the higher-than-average expectations, the burden of dust in her private parts and the inexcusable physical and verbal abuse hurled in her direction. Always trying her best to do her utmost. Countless trips to the doctors to inject extra RAM, eliminate a virus, or simply clean, and she would always return with an earnest zest to work harder and longer.

It is quite an odd feeling when you finally decide to farewell one innate object for a new shiny one. Whilst quite irrational, there is a slight sense of betrayal. You have entered the world of consumerism, and your decision to upgrade needs to be absolutely essential, or is that just me? The payoff, of course, is the nightmare that is currently consuming my time. Setting up 'Bertha' requires the patience and composure of a Zen master. Failing to fall into that category ultimately means that I and anyone in the near vicinity are suffering from upgrade remorse.

The first hurdle is locating the box marked 'computer stuff'. Well, actually, questioning whether or not such a box even exists is the very first issue. Okay, there is a box with various tangled cords, old unlabeled CDs, antiquated floppy disks, empty boxes that once housed something important and multiple manuals, including one for Windows 95. So I finally put power into Bertha, and voila, she comes to life and starts to speak. I listen intently and go through every possible set-up situation. Now it starts getting tricky as she insists on knowing passwords, license keys and ID codes. Finally, after many challenging hours, I can happily declare that the printer now works!

It isn't all bad news for Lola; she hasn't been thrown on the hard waste just yet. The thing is, Lola, contains so much vital information that appears to be in a foreign language to Bertha. The copious copies of photos, scans and documents could be lost forever if she actually said her final shutdown. So whilst she is ancient and slow, her memory is still required to function. I was going through such old files and came across some beautiful memories of Harry's early years, and one such treasure was correspondence to and from Warren Brown.

Harry was seven when Warren Brown, a cartoonist for a major Sydney newspaper and a renowned history buff, released his documentary on the re-enactment of the Peking to Paris race. The 1907 Peking to Paris car rally covered a distance of approximately 14,000 km. Crazy conditions challenged them then, and in 2005, Warren and four other teams tackled the same route in the same make of vintage cars. For some inexplicable reason, Harry took a liking to this documentary and watched it countless times. He drew pictures of the vehicles, including a 1907 Spiker, a 1907 De Dion-Bouton, and a 1907 Itala. With Harry's permission, I sent them to Warren along with a note explaining a little about Harry's own challenges and how he was clearly somewhat obsessed.

Just over a week passed before Harry received the most fantastic parcel. Warren wrote back to Harry and included the Peking to Paris book, his antique compass, and a blue silk scarf. Along the journey, when they crossed into Mongolia, they were greeted by locals who performed a dance. The women had blue silk scarves and gave them to the teams as good luck. Warren gave one of these scarves to Harry.

For years, Harry used this scarf as his own 'good luck' aid, and he still treasures it today. I was flabbergasted then, and re-reading the correspondence again, I am still blown away with genuine admiration for Warren Brown.

Some pretty amazing legends are walking among us mere mortals.

Lola has indeed earned her right to sit quietly in the corner and remind me of the past every now and then.

So there you go…

Thank you so much for your wonderful drawings! I loved your drawing of the Spyker - it was very, very colourful and looked just like the real thing!!
I like drawing trains too — when I was your age, I would draw steam trains like this…

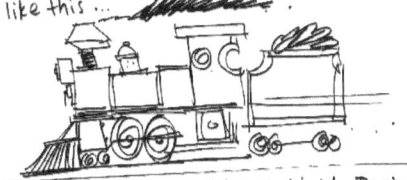
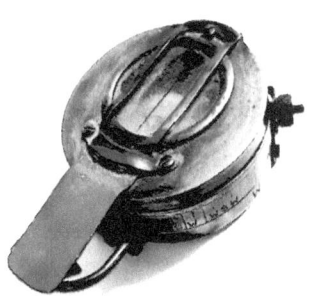

I am so happy you liked Peking to Paris —
To answer your questions —
Paris is a very beautiful city. Very colourful, with lots of great sticky and sweet things to eat. There are hundreds of cars and motorbikes too. I hope you get to see it one day!
When we were in the Gobi Desert, it was cold! Hard to believe isn't it?
It is actually very high above some mountains and very, very, dry. There is no water there at all — (and we were all a bit scared).
I've packed you a blue scarf from Mongolia — it will bring you good luck.
And a copy of our book.
I'm going to send Stynus (the man who drove the Spyker) your drawing of his car. I've also put in a special brass compass so you won't get lost in the Gobi!
Keep in touch!
WARREN (OF PEKING)

TO SAY OR NOT TO SAY

Harry played competitive tennis in his youth. When the Saturday morning scurries of transportation, scorecards, balls and racquets were all sorted, it was time to sit back and watch. One day, I began chatting to the mum of an opposition player. Her name was Kate.

On this occasion, the conversation almost immediately turned to the topic of cancer. The giveaway signature headscarf and weary pallid expression suggested that she was experiencing an illness. From my own experience, I appreciate that people don't always know what to say or how to ask, so I simply inquired if she was okay. I was in my wig phase, so perhaps not so obvious, but maybe there is some sort of cancer radar that those of a feather detect.

Instant simpatico connections are woven from the tapestry of cancer.

Kate had ovarian cancer and had one more round of chemo before tests would determine the outcome. She freely began to unload about her current struggles. Her treatment had seen her hospitalised for periods when her body was unable to handle the effects. She was concerned that the impending results wouldn't match her high expectations. She didn't know how to cope if they didn't, and currently couldn't work - the bills were adding up. She apologised for unloading but felt comfortable talking to someone who may understand. I am very familiar with cancer conversations, and they often seem to go hand in hand with the amount of time spent in the oncology waiting rooms.

Just as with the discussion with Kate, over the years, I have found myself doing more listening than discussing. Perhaps because I have realised that my advanced cancer prognosis is not favourable, and so I hesitate to explain, especially if reassurance is needed. And I have also learnt that comparing cancer diagnoses is not wise, nor necessary, simply because the upshot is so individual. But, still, the need to unburden is perhaps easier within the cancer community. This familiarity led the discussion into that very topic. What *not* to say.

We had both experienced conversations where curious comments had been voiced, but that really just emphasised the many factors and faces of cancer. It has nothing to do with any ill intentions; it is just that sometimes people don't know how to handle it. It's a tricky one because, on the one hand, you don't want people to walk on eggshells and ignore the issue, and on the other, some comments leave you flummoxed. Kate discussed some of the comments that annoyed her…

'*We all have to die of something,*' and '*it could be worse,*' and '*you've got this.*' In the early days, the ones about positivity used to irritate me. '*If anyone is going to get through this, you will.*' It sounds very supportive and helpful; however, I thought I had to retain that image when I didn't feel particularly optimistic. It added pressure. Some have commented. '*What choice do you have? You either get on with it or give up.*' All very pragmatic and logical, but again, there were times when the weight of cancer was unbearable. Sometimes, people wanted to be encouraging and hopeful, but it often came across as dismissive. You don't need a cheerleader or someone solving problems, just someone who pays attention.

I remember discussing how knowing when your time was up would enable you to '*put your house in order*' instead of the inconvenience of dying suddenly. I understand the logic and practicalities in that thought; however, that would also require me to accept that death was my only outcome. Kate said that one of her friends constantly offered, 'If there is anything I can do, just ask.' She understood it was a very kind gesture, but she didn't know how to ask, so she didn't. Her final chemo was approaching, and some of her friends were organising a celebration. So she was anticipating putting on her happy face even though she still felt wary and apprehensive.

I have never really thought it was my place to educate on such matters as what not to say, and so usually just let it go. It is difficult because, like many things, cancer is such an individual experience. What I feel and how I respond or react to anything, including what people say or don't say, can be the complete opposite of someone else.

I do recognise that my opinions have changed over the years. The comments that used to annoy me in the earlier days have little effect now. If someone thinks I'm optimistic, then that's great. I am fortunate to be a positive type of person. Perhaps advanced cancer gives you the gift of a more self-assured perspective, which in turn leads you to conclude that comments simply don't matter.

The conversation then changed direction. Soon after that, Harry's team won the match; we wished each other all the best and went our separate ways. I sometimes wonder what happened to Kate.

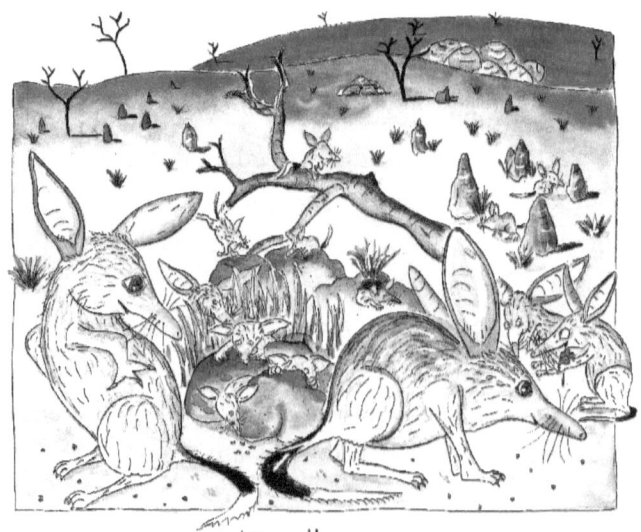

I'm all ears

Wednesdays with Harry
THE BUZZ WORD

Do you ever wonder what happens during your slumber that affects your mood for the day?

My sleep routine is generally less than ideal. If bladder-challenged dogs are not waking me, then I am being transported psychologically (and perhaps physically) into wild and imaginative dreams. It is indeed exhausting surviving a treacherous encounter with a gang of sea monkeys when attempting to be the first woman to sail solo around the world on a banana skin. The ocean is composed of port wine jelly, the oars are hula hoops, the sails are full-brief knickers, and the struggle is real. To the right is Ibis Island, the habitat of five thousand and thirty-two Straw-necked Ibis scavengers and where a volcano of spewing molten lunch wrappers erupts into the sea. To the left, a buzzing reverberation is a squadron of mosquitoes with malicious intent, bearing down and about to attack.

Here it is. Now is the moment when reality interrupts, at first somewhat vaguely, but then quickly with the full force of reality. I find myself with one foot still sailing on the banana skin and the other stepping outside my dream as I realise there was one very determined mosquito targeting my face. It eludes my sleepy objections with stealth and cunning attributes and confidently buzzes louder as it darts towards its prize. I am now fully awake, cursing the mosquito's existence and find myself trying to out-think the predator by wrapping my doona tighter and hitting myself violently in the head. The buzzing is momentarily silenced, and I cautiously rejoice in my victory. However, my experience suggests that one can never be entirely confident that the mosquito will be discouraged. Sure enough, it strikes again, this time from the other direction and with greater noise and determination. Thrashing wildly about and blindly slapping myself in the head was clearly no deterrent for this bloodsucking assassin. Finally, the buzzing subsides, and my bruised and battered body can sink back into slumber. However, it is a restless sleep as I despairingly and drowsily scratch my little finger - the bastard!

I have concluded that mosquitoes are one of the deadliest creatures in the world, not only for their ability to spread infection and disease but also for causing self-inflicted head wounds. I discussed this with Harry. He admits that sleeping for him means entering a world of complete and utter comatose oblivion and has yet to awake for anything, and certainly not for the likes of a tiny pest.

I am now about to spray a suitably toxic chemical throughout the bedroom in the hope that it will obliterate my enemy and create a barrier for blissful sleep.

So there you go…

> If you think you are too small to make a difference, try sleeping with a MOSQUITO!
>
> Dalai Lama

HAZCHEM

April 1986. The Chernobyl nuclear accident is considered to be the worst nuclear disaster in history. Deaths from the immediate accident were reported at thirty-one, but of course, the long-term ramifications were enormous. In 2005, the World Health Organisation estimated five million people still lived in contaminated areas. Four thousand cases of thyroid cancer were linked directly to radiation exposure. Reports from the most affected countries, Russia, Belarus, and Ukraine, differ. Still, it was reported that in 2018, 1,800,000 people in Ukraine, including over 377,000 children, had the status of victims of the disaster. In 2005, it was estimated that between 112,000 and 125,000 people had died. Besides cancers and illness, the rise in suicide, alcoholism and mental health issues has also been attributed to the outcome. It was assessed that five per cent of the nuclear matter leaked into the atmosphere, and strong winds pushed radioactive fallout into Western Europe and Scandinavia. WHO calculated that twenty thousand square kilometres of Europe were contaminated. Plants and grasslands as far away as Britain were polluted, restricting the sale of lamb and sheep products there for years. It is predicted that areas close to the fallout will remain uninhabitable for thousands of years. Needless to say, the accident shocked the world.

At the time, I was working for Contiki Tours, and on April 26th 1986, I was in Oslo, Norway. The seriousness of this news infiltrated the usual laid-back nature of tours. The non-stop party-type hype promised to the eighteen- to thirty-five-year-old crowd stalled for a moment to acknowledge the tragedy and reassess how the tours would proceed. The Russia/Scandi tours were altered to become extended Scandinavian tours, where Vikings and Norwegian trolls leapt into action. We were informed by head office that fresh produce should be avoided at all costs. Many passengers became concerned about their health and left the tours to return home, along with future passengers who cancelled. I am unsure whether the news was reported with less impact in Europe than elsewhere, or if simply existing in our tourism bubble left us ignorant and naive. Except for using long-life milk and eliminating fresh fruit and vegetables, our lives pretty much returned to as before.

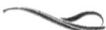

I have never felt why me or questioned how I came to have cancer. It is, however, a requirement when documenting medical information that the family history of cancers is included. My grandfather survived bowel cancer, and my Mum's mother died of ovarian cancer when Mum was in her early teens. My sisters were tested for the BRCA gene to ascertain if there was a genetic link. Fortunately, there was no connection. I completely understand the need to try to find a reason, especially if it is of genetic origin. It can serve as a warning for a family to follow, and it was vital in my own treatment. My parents, however, have often questioned it, and one of their conclusions is my time in Oslo in 1986. I have and still do dismiss this notion. I feel for the multitudes it has so severely affected; however, I wasn't one of them. I view my cancer as crappy bad luck. I appreciate why a parent is more earnest in finding a reason, searching for answers, and hunting down the culprit who has dared to harm their child. Perhaps directing that frustration and anger at something specific is somehow helpful. I, on the other hand, find acceptance a more beneficial emotion.

Now speaking of radiation... The process leading up to having radiotherapy included mapping the area of my chest that was going to be zapped. It was important that when the radiation was shooting into my body, the affected area was precisely the same each time. Therefore, small dots are tattooed on my chest - X marks the spot.

The discussion with the radiotherapist was similar to other consultations, where it was noted how unlucky I was that such a small amount of cancer had caused so much damage. Side effects were explained, along with the usual warnings about potential permanent damage. It was also noted that other cancers can be a result of this treatment. There was no doubt that when you are presented with a room that houses a big three-pronged radioactive sign on the door, it is time that you sit up and take notice of what is in the fine print. It was made very clear that it is entirely your choice to proceed. Did I have a choice, though? At the time, I didn't feel I did, so I agreed to continue.

Every day for the next seven weeks, I drove to the radiation clinic and changed into my gown in preparation for the reasonably short amount of time it took to complete this treatment. I had had enough of struggling into hospital gowns, so I chose to bring my own. It was a lovely floral number, and whilst more attractive and certainly more comfortable, I haven't been able to wear it again since.

Due to other patients being on simultaneous schedules, it was natural to chat or nod in recognition of the familiar. There was an understanding that whilst the areas being treated may differ, essentially, we were all on the same quest. It didn't seem intrusive to be asked which body part would be zapped, and further cancer discussions came with ease. I recall one elderly chap showed clear evidence that his nose was being treated, and unfortunately, the effects were unavoidably visible. I quietly felt gratitude that it wasn't me.

The treatment was a relatively quick process, so waiting was minimal for once. When called, I would chat briefly to the staff whilst assuming my motionless position on the table. A heavy jelly pad thingy was placed on top of my breast area. Staff would then hike it out of there, finding refuge in the adjacent control room, safe from the flexible arm of the linear accelerator and its cancer-zapping radiation beam.

It didn't hurt. Well, I say it didn't hurt; that is, up until the last two weeks. Unfortunately, my chest, inside and out, was starting to suffer from the treatment.

It is hard to know if the future pain, spasms, and inflammation, along with thyroid cancer, resulted from radiotherapy.

I still have the scars and burn marks today.

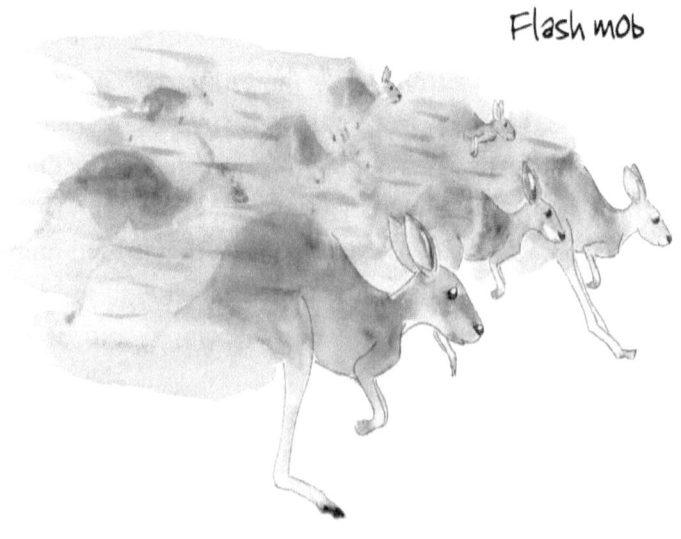

Flash mob

Wednesdays with Harry
REDWOODS

Okay, well, in just over a month, Harry will be twenty-one years of age, so the topic of what he would like as a gift has been broached. Various ideas have been suggested, and the latest is a camera. I explained my concern that he hadn't shown any great interest in photography in the past, and that it might be overlooked due to the convenience of his phone. I suggested that he make use of my camera first to see if the impulse subsided. I then explained my love for photography and how I used to spend hours in my darkroom, wholly absorbed in the process of developing film into negatives and then the anticipation as I swished chemicals over the paper, and miraculously, an image would appear.

I was only equipped to tackle black and white, so the need to develop colour photos professionally was often. To the 'HAVE IT RIGHT NOW' generation, it is difficult to explain or indeed for them to understand that the process from film to photo was a lengthy and expensive one. The first decision was the length of the film, with options of twelve, twenty-four, or thirty-six pictures allowed, and this was the first expense. Harry looked confused. You took your time to take a picture, as there were no 'delete' or 'try again' buttons. Still baffled. If you had an SLR camera, as I did, you needed to understand focusing, depth of field, aperture, and other related concepts. You then send your film off to be developed after proudly assuring yourself that your photographic ability could see you working for National Geographic. You wait patiently for a few days, and then, as expectations of brilliance rise, you open the packet of photos, only to be hit by reality: that sinking feeling when you discover you had just paid for thirty-six photos that highlighted the details of your thumb. Harry's reaction to my musings was in keeping with his usual response - a little confused with superior indifference.

So anyway, back to today's activity. We again kept it in the vicinity of home and took a short drive to the Redwood Forest in East Warburton. Yes, we have visited in the past, but it is an ideal spot for Harry to try out the camera. On the way there, the conversation turned to Harry's choice of clothing. We seem to have had quite a few discussions regarding Harry's clothing on these outings. Today was no exception. Whilst it's only March, the weather was a little cool, so I donned a jumper. Harry, on the other hand, was in a T-shirt. He casually mentioned that we couldn't stay too long, as he was cold and also hungry. I asked him why he didn't seem capable of ascertaining the correct clothing for the weather. He informed me that firstly, it was not winter, so no jumper should be needed, and secondly, the forecast was for twenty-two degrees, both of which meant a T-shirt would be sufficient. I suggested that in future, he simply look outside.

The Redwood Forest is indeed a unique and calming place, with trees stretching straight and skyward, standing in rigid, uniformed rows, with only their canopy allowed to sway. Their strength is comforting. It used to be only locals who knew of its existence. Now the knowledge is spread globally, and tourists gather to partake in her spirit. Today, however, there were very few visitors: a family playing and frolicking in the woven wooden nests, a couple solemnly strolling with contemplation, and Harry and I with photographic intentions.

We ventured past the forest boundary towards the sound of Cement Creek. Harry was quite keen to show that he could master the camera and focused on fungi, ferns and frogs and showed a liking for lichen, leaves and logs. This was, of course, until he explained that his hunger pains were going to 'literally' kill him unless we found food.

You will be pleased to know that I managed to forage for some nourishment just in time, and he is still alive and kicking!

So there you go…

PS: Harry eventually concluded that a sports watch would be more beneficial than a camera. One that not only announced the time but was also programmed to calculate fitness, heart rates, stress levels, music, the NASDAQ, tidal patterns and full moons. It could make a bed, clean the car, predict the lotto numbers and take the dog for a walk…and it glowed in the dark. Voila!

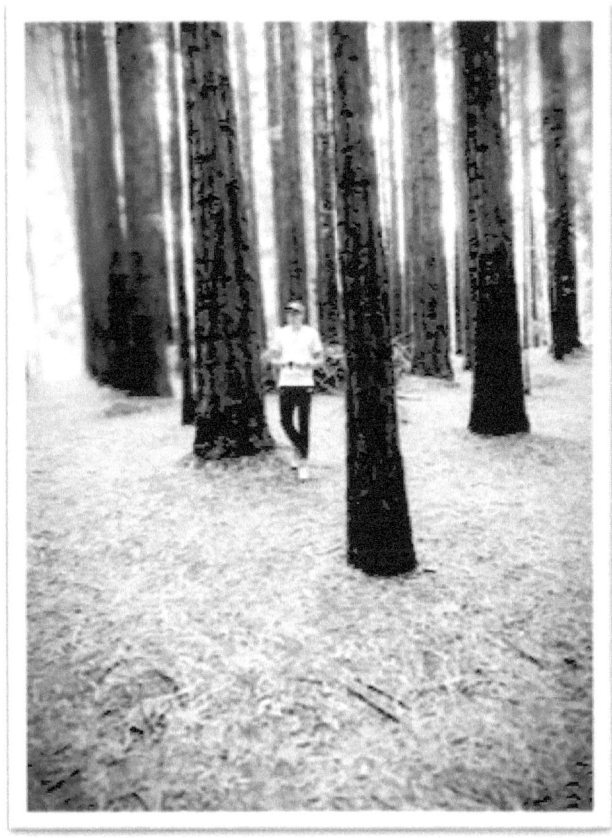

WHAT ABOUT ME?

Jim Stynes passed away from melanoma cancer in March 2012. He was 45.

Jim was a Melbourne Football Club player and president, an AFL Hall of Famer, and a Brownlow medallist, one of the highest football awards. He had a well-celebrated football career; however, he was equally revered for his work outside of football. In 1994, Jim established the not-for-profit Reach Foundation, which supports and inspires young people to make the most of their lives. He announced his cancer diagnosis in 2009 and became a symbol of hope when he continued to show strength and courage in the face of many operations, and when his cancer metastasised to his brain. He let the public in and allowed us to witness his confrontation with cancer. We held him up on a pedestal of heroism and declared our full support. We urged him to keep fighting and felt the impact when setbacks occurred. His death touched not only those in the sporting world but also the broader community.

I remember at the time, someone created controversy by questioning the need for a State funeral. He declared that, while Jim was a tough and talented footballer who had made significant contributions to society, he thought a State funeral was excessive. He felt that many others contributed to the community and suffered similar journeys, but didn't receive the same attention and recognition. Perhaps his view was affected because he had watched his mother suffer and die from cancer. Many declared their horror at his attitude, and he soon apologised and indicated that his comments were not clearly understood.

This has been an opinion that I have wondered about from time to time. Not regarding this personal reference to Jim Stynes or the abysmal timing and point of someone's comments, but regarding the varying degree of value we put on lives, particularly comparing with those who are in the public eye. Is there any difference? Do we really believe that someone recognised or famous has a different cancer experience than anyone else? Being witness to a publicly recognised personality in their cancer struggle and suffering does allow creating awareness and education where otherwise perhaps ignorant. Inspiration is also a relevant term tossed about and can truly put our own lives into perspective.

Perhaps the select few benefit from gaining empathy, sympathy, and support from the masses. Swaddled and comforted when times are tough from multitudes of admirers, I can imagine, would be heartening. However, regardless of the amount of outpouring and support, it could not fill the lonely void that comes with facing your own mortality.

Cheryl, a woman I met in oncology in 2012, gravely ill with advanced breast cancer, was no less deserving of all the love and attention offered to prominent others. Her quiet grace and acceptance of what was coming her way was only noted and felt by those closest to her. But that was okay because the thing is - whether someone has thousands of well-wishers or simply a few close friends, for both, it is a solitary walk to the end.

I think that whether someone is honoured with a State funeral fanfare or not is totally irrelevant to the essence of someone's life. Comparing your life with someone famous, or in fact, anyone else, and then asking *'what about me?'* is simply futile.

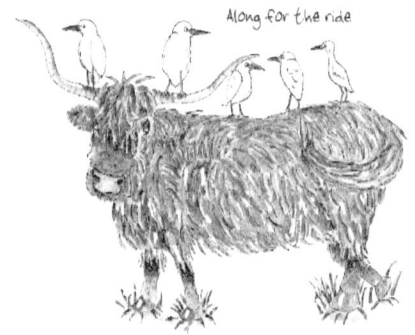
Along for the ride

Wednesdays with Harry
ANZAC DAY

Anzac Day in Australia and New Zealand is by far the most significant day when we pause to remember and honour those who have served. Thankfully, we had moved past the times when protests marred the day. There will likely be those who attempt to compare its significance to other issues. It doesn't need to be compared.

'ANZAC is not a place or a time – it is a bond of people and a legacy we continue'.

The alarm was set for 4:00 am. Dragging Harry out of bed before daybreak to attend the dawn service at the Shrine indeed tested his value of such an occasion. Sleep versus partaking in life's events is always a question that often sees sleep as the victor. Fortunately for Harry, however, he has a mum who nags, pokes, prods, persists and insists that he rise from his slumber and attend such a ceremony.

We managed to overcome early morning challenges such as inserting contact lenses and finding matching socks, and gradually gained some perspective on the significance of such a day.

Thousands of people came from all directions, walking solemnly yet proudly, drawn magnetically towards the beacon on the hill - The Shrine. There is a feeling of solidarity in the dark; the acceptance of bonding is evident with strangers silently acknowledging the reason we congregate on this day, at this hour.

Harry did wonder why we were standing among a crowd of thirty-five thousand so early. I calmly explained that the clue was in the title: 'dawn service.'

Observing the crowd, it was easy to see the various levels of the dawn service experience. Some knew that bringing a chair and a thermos was part of the ritual, while novices like us just stood with aching calves, wishing we were better prepared.

The waiting begins. Quiet reflection is periodically interrupted by the snapping of photos and the cramping of toes.

When the ceremony comes to life, we hear about individuals and groups who have experienced what no person should. Some make it home to tell the stories, and others give the ultimate sacrifice. We listen to *"In Flanders Fields "* and try to gain insight. The emotion spreads throughout the crowd.

The Last Post is always a teary, significant and final moment. Played by a lone bugler seems somewhat appropriate and, for me, the most poignant part of the ceremony.

Australia doesn't always get it right – but on this day, I think we do.

So there you go...

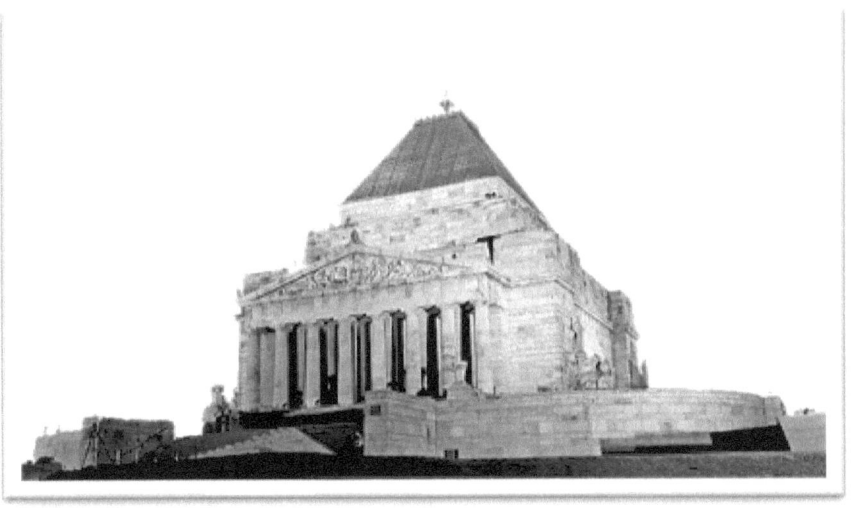

HEADSPACE HERO

Every now and then, you connect with a person, a theory, an idea, or a belief, and voilà, suddenly a rocky path is illuminated with strategy and clarity. For Harry, and in extension, myself, it was Nick Duigan.

As already noted, Harry had anxiety challenges in his youth, and it was clear that professional help was needed. During his younger years, he did see various specialists; however, the clinical nature of medical offices only added to his apprehension. The fact that he was a tad obsessed with football, and particularly the Carlton Football Club, turned out to be the catalyst for a relationship that could finally make a difference. What are the odds that an AFL footballer was a qualified psychologist AND played for Carlton? Besides fiercely running amok on the half-back line, Nick Duigan worked as a clinical psychologist and really had little choice but to take Harry on as a client. At last, I could pry Harry out of the car and into the multifaceted world of psychology.

One of the most significant theories Nick imparted is called ACT, or Acceptance and Commitment Therapy. In many ways, I think I have always naturally gravitated towards such ideas, but the introduction to it as an actual structured theorem was enlightening. Put simply, it is using mindfulness as a tool to overcome anxiety. The concept of 'acceptance' is about accepting things just the way they are, whether good or bad. It's not about eliminating stress; it's about acknowledging it and finding ways to manage it. 'Give me the courage to accept the things I cannot change…'

Identifying your values is vital as they enable motivation to change your life for the better. Of course, it isn't enough to simply discuss such ideas; you need to put in the work and complete the exercises. Using diffusion or distraction techniques to lessen the impact of painful or powerful thoughts becomes such an important tool and has indeed been a saviour to both Harry and me. Harry was armed with affirmations that confirmed these ideas, and he regularly repeated them. For example, 'thoughts cannot hurt me, they are just like clouds, and they come and go all by themselves.'

Mindfulness is simply the practice of being completely present. So, from learning the mindful body scan to mindfully eating a mandarin, Nick gently guided Harry through the exercises, and in turn, Harry was able to achieve a great deal. When the world was closing in, he could stand on the balls of his feet, pause and notice how that physically felt. Everything else faded into the background, allowing his mind to slow down and be present. Recognising when you have a powerful thought is not easy, as we tend to react quickly. Still, exercises such as rating the impact on a scale and then singing that same formidable thought or perhaps saying it in a different voice really do have an effect. Harry's go-to voice of choice was Frank Walker from National Tiles, and I can assure you the weight of that thought disappeared immediately. Ultimately, you cannot change what you think or feel, but you can work on how you react.

Nick challenged Harry with so many ideas, and Harry responded. Nick was most likely one of the most significant influences in Harry's young life, and he will perhaps never really realise the impact he had. And I, in turn, have the most tremendous respect.

These tools have also been of enormous help to me. I recall my first MRI experience. I was a little concerned, not only about the impending results but also about the claustrophobic conditions that may prove difficult. So, in preparation, I decided to lie back, close my eyes, and visualise the entire *Sound of Music* movie. Sorry to say that the lonely goatherd stayed high on the hill, as I didn't realise that I would be required to work during this procedure and was kept busy breathing in and out when requested. Also, the jackhammer noise that accompanied the machine was a bit of a killjoy to my rendition of

Do-Re-Mi. Either way, I was distracted and sailed through it unscathed.

Nowadays, I use it constantly for both big and small stuff, from feeling annoyed at traffic to waiting for test results. Knowing that thoughts cannot hurt me, diffusing the power of thoughts and staying present have all been so beneficial. When life is consumed with anxiety and fear, I can guarantee that singing the thought, '*I'm going to die from cancer,*' in the voice of Kermit the Frog, really does quieten the noise.

Thanks Nick.

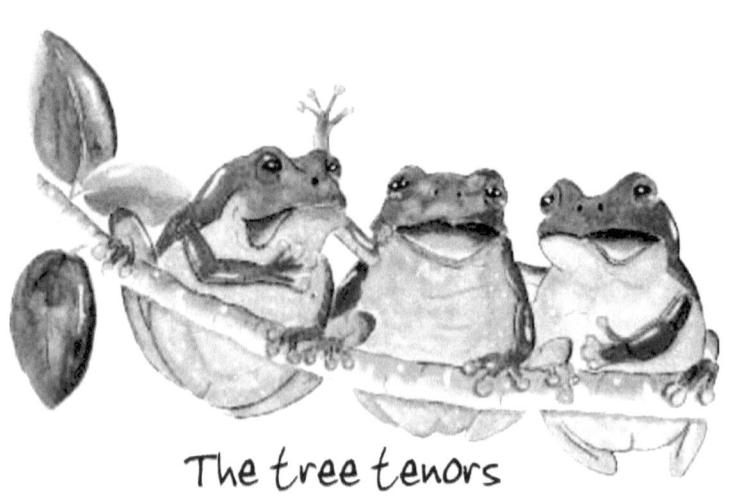

The tree tenors

Wednesdays with Harry
SPLITTING HAIRS

It is a requirement that Harry gain a student card for University. Of course, as a photo would be imprinted on the card, the same one for several years, it was important to Harry that it was an acceptable one. Personally, as someone who dislikes having my photo taken and displayed in any format, I can understand his thinking.

It was always very evident that Harry's hair DNA came from me – very thick and fast-growing - well, for me that was BC (before chemo). Therefore, the need for frequent hair clipping has always been an issue. This situation meant that the desire for a good photo with a half-decent haircut was in direct conflict with the tiresome process of having said haircut. Just as I thought, however, the photo won, and so it was off to find a talented barber or hairdresser who could cut just the correct number of hairs.

We decided that Chadstone Shopping Centre, quite possibly the largest shopping complex on earth, would indeed house this gifted coiffeur who would be able to take up the challenge.

Speaking of challenges, finding a car park was the first one. Success was on the verge, but alas, many attempts trawling multiplex car parks resulted in failure, and ongoing disappointment ensued. Your heart skips a beat when you're teased with the one rare green light, beckoning an end to this car-parking trauma by indicating a vacant spot. You cunningly outwit other vehicles to hunt it down, only to find it housed a trolley bay, a disabled park or simply a malfunction. The initial positive mood quickly drains away, and you start to question the need for this entire expedition. Finally, you turn into a row where a mother, mustering three kids whilst pushing an overloaded trolley, is heading for her car. You appear to have no other choice but to sit and wait, blinker on, with full indicator contractual rights that you have dibs on this park. The time it takes for her shopping to be unloaded, the kids to be organised, and the trolley to be returned is agonisingly slow. Then, before leaving, she appears to check her texts and clearly needs to reply with a thousand-word essay. At this point, you begin to cry, and any remaining enthusiasm for this task has been completely extinguished.

So, finally we parked, but finding a hairdresser proved to be yet another challenge. Locating and then utilising the vital information display board system was another test. I proceeded to type and enter the category hairdressers. Harry's patience with my understanding of how such a screen should work was tested, and it wasn't long before he took over the task. For future reference, hairdressers are not listed under 'B' for Beauty, as Harry assumed - astonishingly enough, they are listed under 'H' for Hairdressers.

So, we picked a possible winner and then, of course, had to work out the map to locate the chosen salon. Unfortunately, neither of us could actually remember more than twenty metres of the map before we had to refer to another information board again. Argh! I am, however, pleased to announce that we eventually found a first-rate stylist who met Harry's specific hairstyle requirements.

We then found ourselves in that time-vacuum of shopping. You know, it is where one becomes oblivious to outside obligations and therefore confidently ambles about with the impulsive mindset of *'since we are here, we may as well...'* Blissfully ignorant of actual schedules and dangerously abusing time. Before we knew it, we had to get to the University pronto if Harry was to have his student card processed and be back in time for footy training. Therefore, the pace was lifted. Harry's encouragement of my walking speed was a mix of desperation, stress, and frustration.

Eventually, the escalator was one of the last obstacles between us and the car park. Harry managed to weave a path past languid shoppers who were haphazardly littered along the moving staircase. His utterance of '*We're not all here for a ride*' was clearly meant for all to hear.

So, we made it to the Uni, trawled another car park, navigated another map and discovered the Student Central Centre is in building HE. I suggested that he smile pleasantly for his photo.

'*Mum, smiling is a sign of weakness,*' he explained. Of course!

Finally, the mission was accomplished - AND we made it back in time for training.

So there you go...

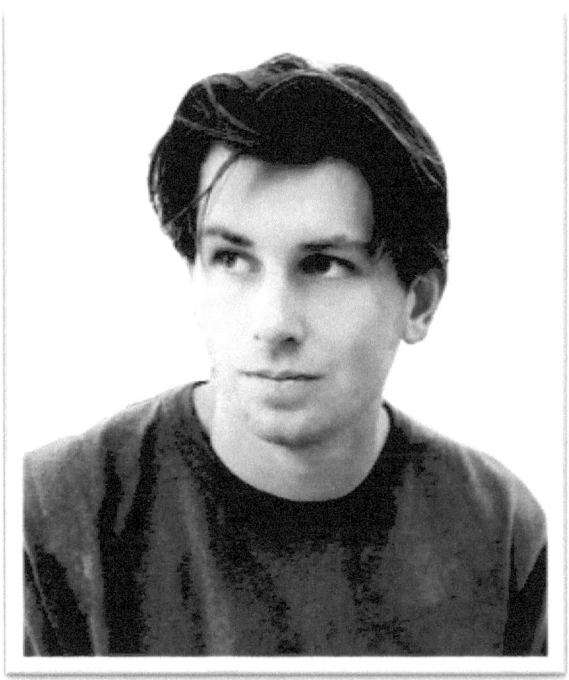

THE CLINIC
December 13th, 2013

A sudden rush of dread overwhelms me as I approach the door to the breast clinic. It has been almost three years since my first appointment, but with every visit, the apprehension remains. I know that sometimes it is simply my mind recalling the first time. The first time I was at the clinic to await my fate. '*My life is about to change forever,*' strung on a banner across my thoughts. Now with every visit, that same banner flies in the shadows of my mind, always with that fundamental niggling question...

Today, I entered the clinic, and the familiar surroundings helped ease my concerns. The woman on reception immediately recognises me and offers the usual friendly greeting. We chat briefly about the glorious sunny day whilst my attendance is processed before being directed to the waiting room. The room has about twelve seats, and all but two are taken. I settle into the chair in the corner and know that, like most visits, the wait could be lengthy. I take out my phone and fiddle with some buttons, attempting to be interested in something other than why I am here. It doesn't take long for me to start casually glancing around the room. The magazine table is strewn with current news and old stories, and I am sitting next to the bookshelf where Dan Brown and Dick Frances novels dominate the shelves. I notice the same tired décor. The familiar patchwork quilt hung on a wall that someone had lovingly toiled over, explicitly themed with breast cancer symbols. On the adjacent wall is the mandatory Monet print in a faded silver frame. Hanging off the curtain pelmet is a gold metallic angel, a new addition, another symbol. The final embellishment is an inspirational cross-stitch, 'May every hour give hope, every week give strength and every year courage.' The pamphlet rack is neatly filled with information on every conceivable cancer subject. Escape is impossible.

I had now been waiting about ten minutes, long enough to allow me to shift my glance and observe others in the room. Most are here as couples. The bloke on my right is slumped in his chair and appears to be taking a nap. I suspect, however, he may have finished reading the sporting section of the paper and closing his eyes is the best choice to pass the time. His partner is looking annoyed. A mother and daughter are present, and I quickly ascertain that the mother is the patient. A young couple struggling to feed their infant child allows a break in the silence. For a brief time, the child provides some welcome distraction. I wonder if the child will ever come to know the impact of that waiting room, and pray she doesn't need to.

It occurred to me that various experiences of cancer were most likely represented in that waiting room. There are the first-timers, anxiously clutching their crisp X-ray envelopes, desperately hoping the contents are benign. The women in the chemo stages of treatment, the scarves and hats are a sure giveaway. The next group consists of more seasoned patients, whose physical scars have healed, and wigs and scarves have been replaced by naturally regrown hair. Finally, there are those who have years of experience. They have an air of confidence, have endured thus far, and wisely bring their knitting. The chances of us all surviving this are slim - will it be me who succumbs? A middle-aged woman sitting across the room from me is looking particularly concerned. I tried to catch her eye with a reassuring smile, but she was too deep in her own thoughts to notice my gaze. I know how worried I was at my initial diagnosis and how no one could have penetrated my catastrophising mind.

One by one, the patients are called, and they follow their doctor to receive their fate.

I recall when I was first diagnosed, exposed, in a daze, with nowhere to hide. You have just been told the most devastating news, and yet find yourself dealing with the reality of organising the next appointment and treatment. I remember standing in line at the reception with a woman who was rejoicing that she had just gone seven years and given the all-clear. Perhaps our mind going into shock is the most helpful way to cope. I was able to function. That experience allowed me the knowledge that one's relief may be entangled with another's disbelief. I remain aware of this situation today.

Finally, I am called. The doctor wastes no time. He begins by searching for my original diagnosis and prognosis. Ah, yes, there we go. He reminds me how unlucky I am with the particularly aggressive nature of my cancer, as if that piece of information may have somehow slipped my mind. Okay, now moving on to the current test results. Deep breath. The biopsy on the growing nodules in my thyroid is indeed cancer, and the thyroid will have to be removed. Another surgeon will be involved, but the good news is that the chance of survival from thyroid cancer is high.

The journey at The Clinic continues.

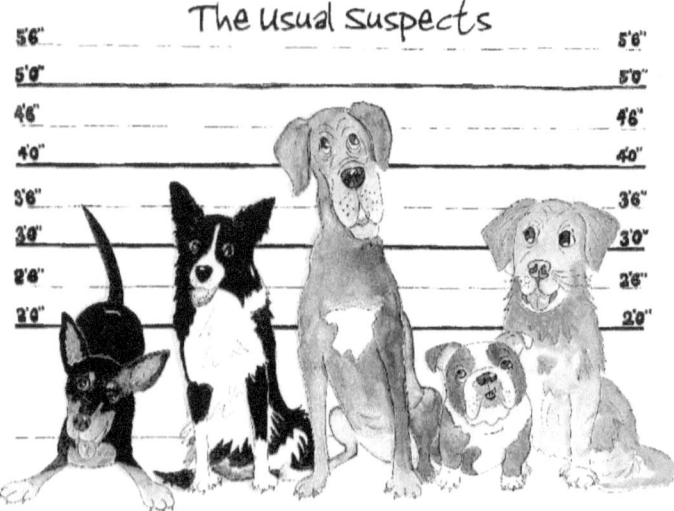

Wednesdays with Harry
DANNY FRAWLEY

September 11th, 2019

It has been quite an emotional week. Perhaps because we are overtired from watching the Ashes cricket all night, but mainly for the passing of Danny Frawley. For many not connected in the AFL football world, his passing may not have triggered such a response, and whilst we didn't know him personally, the tragedy of his death has left a very hollow, shocked and empty feeling.

For Harry, Danny Frawley has been significant in his world for many years. He would always scramble to listen to radio's Triple M Saturday Rub and, in more recent times, would never miss an episode of The Bounce. Of course, it wasn't only Danny's involvement that enticed such an audience; it was the combination of banter among personalities bonded over the sport of AFL football. There is no denying that Danny's contribution to these groups had a huge impact, especially his contagious laugh and sense of humour.

The impact of his death has shattered the football community. Whilst we are a football-loving family, many may not agree, understand, or care about the sport. It is indeed just a game where players run about kicking an odd-shaped ball between two posts. You may dislike the game, be indifferent to the passion that afflicts its supporters, and be utterly bored that it is a topic of conversation that dominates workplaces and public spaces. You may easily conclude that there is more to life than this sport and be totally bamboozled by those who have been taken under its spell. I have no need or desire to change minds on any of that, nor apologise for my love of the game, but I would like to attempt to explain why football is important to us and why the passing of Danny Frawley holds such emotion.

Growing up in a football household meant Saturdays were spent ardently following the team Dad coached and riding the highs and lows, knowing that his contribution positively affected so many. He was involved in junior teams where he could teach kids not just how to play football, but also how to behave. So many years have passed, but countless ex-footballers still have so much respect for Dad. The Carlton Football Club has also been so significant to my family. My father has always been a passionate supporter, and for the past forty-three years, he has also contributed to their recruiting program and is a very proud Life Member. His involvement has given him the most fantastic set of friends and bonds that have lasted a lifetime. It is indeed a family.

I most likely did have a choice regarding the team I supported, but really, why would I choose any team other than Carlton? And I have been fortunate to have witnessed some of the club's most glorious victories. Whilst Harry hasn't been able to enjoy such halcyon days just yet, it was really never in doubt who he would support.

Harry has played footy since the age of seven when Auskick sparked the flame. Playing football has helped him overcome some of his personal hurdles by being accepted as part of a team. The fact that footy has given him a fit and healthy lifestyle, taught him resilience, and social acceptance has been vital in his development.

For me, the positives far outweigh the negatives, and Danny Frawley was the epitome of everything great about the game. Providing young people, particularly young males, with a purpose to be fit, healthy, and a sense of community is a crucial factor. The consequence of the football community using its popularity to educate on racial and gender acceptance, as well as mental health issues, is invaluable.

Danny Frawley's passion for football and his forceful sense of humour attracted so many fans. He reinforced the spirit and promotion of the game in such a likeable fashion.

The shock of Danny Frawley's passing has left us questioning how such a vibrant, passionate and humorous personality could come to the conclusion that he needed to leave this world. It highlights the true ramifications of mental health issues and depression, and how even those surrounded by close mates and who appear able to fight through the fog are left vulnerable to depression's dark spaces. Perhaps his legacy will be this very realisation.

I have had discussions with Harry about how he feels. He is still shocked that this man he revered on many levels is no longer here, but it has opened up dialogue regarding mental health issues among his peers. I can only hope open discussions and awareness will help, and that he never feels so desperately lost and alone.

In my world, the longevity of my own life is challenged, but I am grateful that I have a very strong determination that I will do anything to prolong it. The thought that others choose to leave this world, in my mind, simply cements the understanding that I am the lucky one.

R.I.P. Danny Frawley.

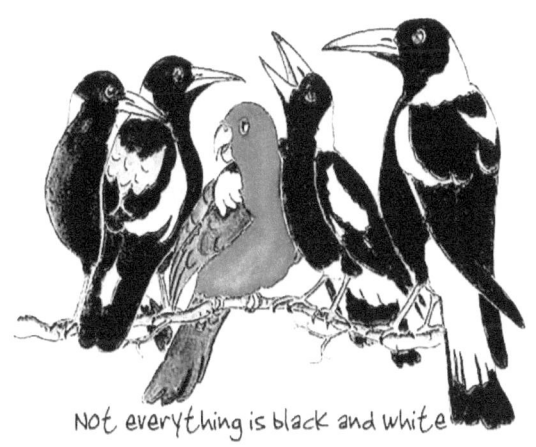

Not everything is black and white

GAME, SET...THYROID

Harry was a keen tennis player in his youth. Lessons led to playing junior competition, and as Warburton is quite a small town, it wasn't surprising that the team was made up of friends from school. They progressed pretty quickly and, over the years, secured many premierships along with becoming great mates. Harry's personality invited him to go all in. Multiple trips to Tennis Warehouse would see him decked out in the latest Federer apparel, overflowing sporting bags with tennis paraphernalia, and adopting a keen interest in all things tennis.

The Australian Open tournament, held annually in Melbourne in January, is an exciting event that Harry craved to participate in. He decided he would be a Ballkid. Thousands applied for approximately 300 positions, making it quite challenging to be selected. The process was lengthy and comprehensive, involving numerous rounds of tryouts and practice sessions over the course of a year. In 2012, Harry made it to the last round before being told he wasn't successful and was advised to try again the following year. Rejection and disappointment didn't deter him, and so, with the understanding and incentive that the Lacoste Ballkid uniform he wore would be his to keep, he gave it another go the following year. After much practice and many training sessions later, he was selected to be an Australian Open Ballkid for the upcoming January tournament.

As already mentioned, anxiety for Harry was something he needed to constantly address. Still, it has always amazed me that his enthusiasm to be selected or involved in any sporting event ran deeper, no matter how overwhelmed he may have felt. With the learned tools in place, he could do anything. Stress is not something that has to be avoided; you just need to know how to handle it.

That December, leading up to the AO, Harry was busy with final training sessions, uniform fittings, and security passes were prepared, as well as rules and procedures were understood.

For me, it was learning I had thyroid cancer.

One of the benefits of being involved in a clinical trial was having an annual MRI on my entire body. In 2012, an abnormality was picked up on my thyroid, and so a biopsy followed. It was benign. Precisely a year later, another MRI showed other nodules in my thyroid, and again, a biopsy was taken. On December 13th, 2013, Mum's birthday, we met the family at a café where we briefly celebrated before I headed off to the breast clinic to learn the results. When the doctor informed me, it was indeed thyroid cancer, my first thoughts were that the breast cancer had metastasised, and I could be in a much crappier situation. I was told that it wasn't related. Just bad luck. Now, where had I heard that before? A trainee doctor was also in attendance and inquired if I had been exposed to any radiation recently. I explained I had radiotherapy two years prior. He quickly changed the subject and then left the room. Of course, that piqued my interest, but no answers were forthcoming. I didn't push it. How it came to be seemed less relevant than what we were going to do about it.

The recommendation was an operation where they would remove only one side of my thyroid to leave me with some resemblance of an endocrine system. I was told they would know after the operation if I needed further treatment, but either way, it was curable. The thought of my throat being incised didn't thrill me too much, nor the idea that I would be on permanent thyroid medication, but besides that, I was okay. I didn't get upset, I didn't feel fear, and I didn't panic or go numb. Now I am willing to concede that my incredibly blasé reaction may have been because a far more serious breast cancer diagnosis had already shocked my world. Therefore, this in comparison was minor. But perhaps it was simply that I was told my thyroid cancer was curable and wouldn't end my life. No drama.

The Australian Open began in mid-January, and with a city apartment secured for the next two weeks, Bryce and I played a tag team to be there when needed for Harry. My operation was scheduled for the Friday of the first week of the competition. I spent the day before at the tennis. The day was sweltering, and the only respite was found in the air-conditioned toilets or in front of the industrial-sized fans provided for their fan-fanning ability. Ballkids and players were dropping like flies. Harry had to fill in for others who had succumbed to the heat. Temperatures during that first week ranged from 41 to 44 degrees. On that Thursday, the play was delayed mid-afternoon and resumed later that evening when the heat lessened. That meant that Harry's session went on into the following morning. Thankfully, we had organised the apartment close by. Whilst I wanted to stay and be a mum, I had no option but to swap with Bryce and take my melted body home in preparation for Friday's op.

I really don't like being in hospital. Love the staff and their dedication and compassion, but everything else is tainted with smells and illness, intrusive motives, communal sharing, dreary colours and tasteless food. The least amount of time I spend in one, the better.

Putting aside the thought that my throat was about to be cut, I sailed into the operation early that morning with quiet resignation. All went well. By mid-afternoon, I was recovering and desperately trying to convince anyone who would listen that I was fine and could go home. Unfortunately, I was staying put.

Now, I don't wish to sound ungrateful for the public health system we are afforded in this country, as we are fortunate to be taken care of regardless of our insurance or wealth, but I do have one gripe. When you are a female and have had bits cut out, sharing a ward, which of course includes toilet facilities, with blokes who are there for infected toes or thrombosed haemorrhoids, is not ideal. And let's not go into the snoring issues. I would have had more rest sleeping in the car park.

Over the years, I can honestly say that I have rarely played the cancer card. I can hardly stand and declare my need for normality and then cry '*but look at me!* 'I don't think feeling sorry for yourself is at all beneficial. However, I will admit that on this occasion, when the yob in the neighbouring bed insisted on telling me his hard-luck story regarding his festering fungal toe, I broke my own rules. At the end of his woeful toe tale, he yelled across to me, '*hey lovey, what ya in fa?*' I simply muttered back in the most pathetic voice, '*cancer*'. '*God, sorry mate*,' came his reply. He then shifted tack and repeated his story to the thrombosed haemorrhoids bloke across the way. The nurses understood and, after that, left my curtains closed.

I convinced the doctor the following day that I was good to go, and so with a scarf carefully placed around my wound, I managed to return to the tennis on Monday. Possibly not recommended, but I felt fine. As it turned out, the cancer was right in the middle of my thyroid, and so a month later, they had to operate again to take the remaining half. So now I live without my thyroid and have since realised that your thyroid gland is quite important. It affects hormones and metabolism, and apparently, thyroid hormones are essential for the function of every cell in the body. Fortunately, we live in a time where medication can simulate its function. Took a bit of adjusting, however. That first year, I managed to pile on an enormous amount of weight simply by staring at lettuce. I also discovered that if the dose isn't quite right, it can cause a chemical imbalance and muck about with your mental health.

Meanwhile, back at the tennis…Harry had a wonderful experience as a Ballkid, and he was also selected the following year. Over the years, I have been extremely proud of Harry, and indeed, how he conducted himself in the lead-up and during the Australian

Open was one of them. I could easily see that many times his apprehensions were massive, but he pushed through and did a great job. He was rewarded for his efforts in his last year by being allocated the men's semi-final on Rod Laver Arena between Andy Murray and Tomas Berdych. The Ballkids schedule was only listed the day prior, so it was a last-minute scramble to secure a ticket for myself. We could only afford one. Friends and family were fixated on their telly that night, not necessarily to watch the match but rather to try and gain a glimpse of Harry. I spent the match madly texting to all in sundry when he was on or off the court, and pretty soon, my enthusiasm for the Ballkids was noticed by those seated nearby. From then on, Section thirty-six, Row GG & part of HH, promptly joined in cheering for Harry with all the excitement and interest of a delighted parent. It was quite a night.

The journey it took for Harry to accomplish such a feat was huge, and he was and is undoubtedly just as gutsy and determined as anyone I have known. Is there such a thing as tears of pride? Still affected today.

By the way, Andy Murray won in four. He was defeated by Djokovic in the final.

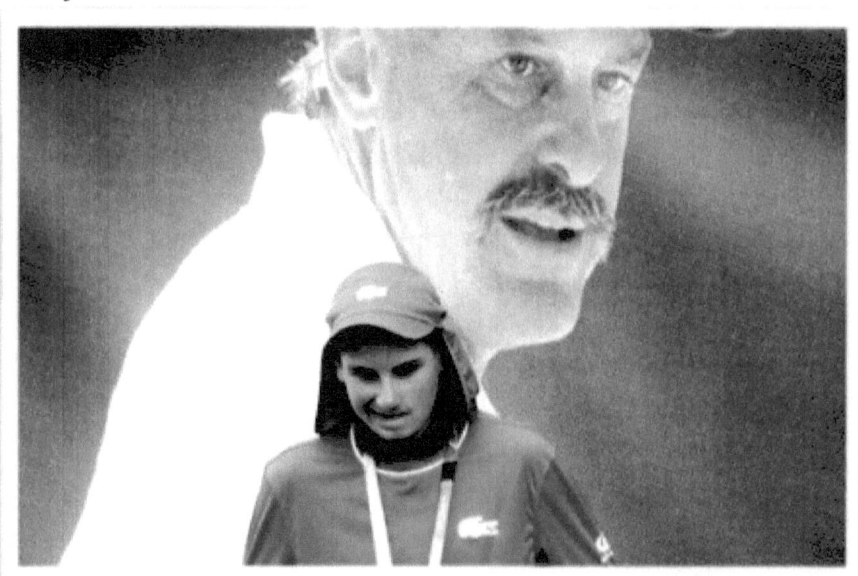

Wednesdays with Harry
FRENCH IMPRESSIONISM

A conspiracy theorist may well believe that the electricity supplier is in cahoots with the National Gallery of Victoria. It does appear that every school holidays, they plan a scheduled power outage, and we find ourselves shuffling through the gallery with perhaps other artificial cultural seekers who cannot seem to last a day without electricity. Of course, for us, this is a two-part equation. The first is that Harry suffers greatly from electricity withdrawal, and the second is that I quite enjoy the gallery. This then combines into an agreeable decision to drive 1.5 hours, (which by the way, is vastly increased by the number of roadworks en route), attempt to park within cooee and then spend the minimum required attendance at the actual gallery.

Speaking of roadworks - in the four times we have been in Covid lockdown over the past year, did it not occur to the roadwork authorities to conduct such maintenance issues DURING this time, when the majority of us were NOT trying to actually USE the roads and advance to our destinations WITHOUT delays?

Masks secured in place and tickets digitally prepared, we strode into the gallery with expectations of enlightenment regarding French Impressionism. No doubt from previous encounters, you do already realise that Harry's expectations are a little different to mine. He is okay with having a gander, a squiz, and a glimpse of what all the fuss is about; however, reading any explanation attached to each painting is pushing it. He manages to take the obligatory photo and shows enough interest to appease me whilst holding onto the knowledge that lunch is imminent.

I may not be the most passionate student of art; however, I do happen to enjoy this particular period, and surprisingly, I was able to pick a Monet from a Manet, a Renoir from a Boudin and a Cezanne from a Sisley. The appreciation of this exhibit from the broad array of visitors seemed genuine. However, I do find that when presented with a 'cultural' experience, there is an underlying pressure to appear educated. One tends to linger and gaze into artwork with perhaps an overzealous enthusiasm, just in case one is mistaken as ignorant. Or maybe one dawdles as they simply want their money's worth? In our case, going to the gallery with Harry certainly ensures that I am not confused about the length of time spent on each painting.

Indeed, art appreciation is an individual quest, and I may never quite understand why the elderly woman wearing a green woollen hat stopped to study a Manet painting for some considerable time. The picture, titled " Street Singer ," illustrates a rather grim-looking lady holding her guitar and eating cherries. Perhaps she was wondering why, when munching on a bunch of cherries, would Manet emulate someone so ashen?

I grew up on a cherry orchard, and I can assure you that each cherry I consumed was a joy. I can clearly recall sitting upon the top of a ladder, bucket belted around my waist and making the tough decisions as a twelve-year-old cherry picker expert was required to do. Should this lustrous, juicy, plump, perfectly formed, delicious red morsel go into the bucket or into my mouth? In those days, the pay was ninety cents per half case, and at that age, that took me about two hours to pick. The decision was easy – into the mouth it went. So, therefore, all I can say about that is that Manet's insight into cherry devouring is very different to mine. Interpretation, conception, perception creates imagination, emotion and thought - and that, my friends, equals art.

The final door led us to the exit via the gift shop, where the artworks were transformed into crockery, tea towels, notebooks, bags and magnets and where I did happen to purchase a print, a Degas, *The Ballet Dancer*.

Much to Harry's disappointment, lunch was somewhat underwhelming, but hey, the power was back on by the time we arrived home, and the exhibit was worth the visit.

So there you go…

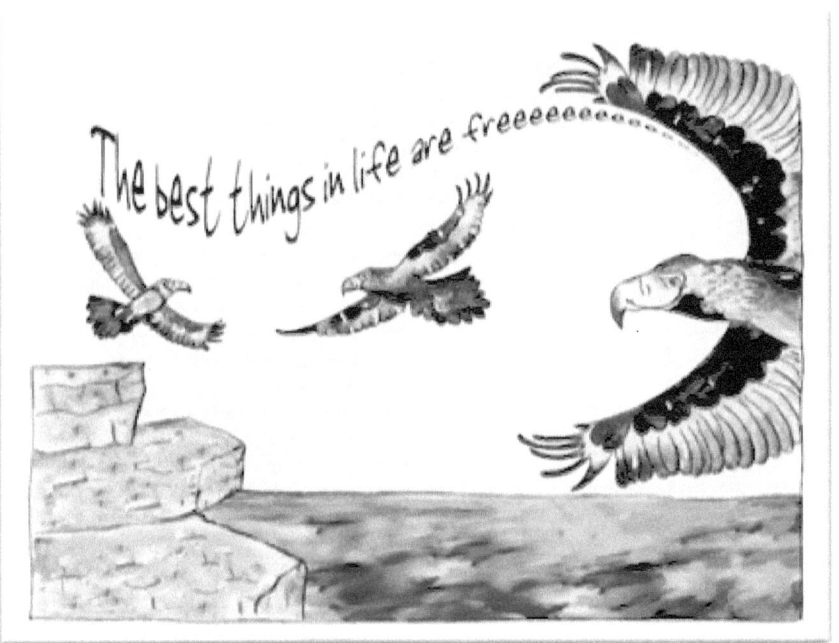

LIVING IN LIMBO

Black Saturday, February 7th 2009. As many as four hundred individual fires were alight across Victoria. The impact caused 173 fatalities – the highest ever loss of human life from bushfires in Australia. The devastation was catastrophic. Further to the human lives lost was the heartbreaking loss of wildlife and the destruction of homes and vegetation. Over 400 people were seriously injured; 1,100,000 acres were burnt; 7562 people were displaced; 3,500 structures were destroyed; over 11,800 livestock perished, and 244,470 acres of national parks were damaged. The number of wildlife that died was overwhelming. The fires raged throughout February and were finally all contained by mid-March.

I remember February 7th clearly. Leading up to the weekend, we were warned that dangerous weather elements were aligned, and potential fire outbreaks were predicted by authorities. As I live in a bushfire area, we are always a little edgy when days like this occur. You prepare as much as possible but know that ultimately you will need to decide to stay or go. You learn to pay attention, as there could very well be a period where it becomes too late to leave. I pray that never happens and feel for those who have had to experience it.

The morning began forebodingly hot, and by mid-morning, the winds were exceeding 100kph. Darkened smoke-filled clouds dominated the skies by late afternoon, and an eerie menacing atmosphere declared the approaching danger. Ash began to fall from the fires raging in the Kinglake area and then from the Marysville fires. It was time to leave. I grabbed Harry, the dogs and a few belongings and drove to my parents. There is really only one road out of our town and traffic was slow. Bryce stayed and was joined by brothers-in-law to make sure live embers didn't ignite a new fire. We were fine.

During the coming weeks, the town was abuzz with activity. Radio stations set up camp in the main street to transmit reports on the latest fire news and attempt to capture the tense atmosphere. The nearby footy oval was the base for the State Emergency Service and firefighting aircraft. Everyone was on tenterhooks, waiting, trapped in limbo and life put on hold. Some seemed to thrive on the excitement, and others were stuck in the headlights. But either way, life was stalled. There were regular meetings organised by the fire authorities to inform residents of the impending threats. Fires were raging in all directions, and we were pretty much surrounded. At one point, we were told that it would likely impact the town within hours, but the weather conditions changed at the last minute. We were still fine.

Those who had to face the actual fire experienced absolute terror, fear, panic, and possible loss of property, injury and life. But we were fine. We only had to contend with the potential threat. We were able to make calm decisions about whether to stay or leave; we had options.

I attended many CFA (Country Fire Authority) meetings over that period and observed signs of outrage, fear and frustration from many residents. Some individuals were struggling to cope with the potential threat, and discussions were often influenced by concern and anger. Many professed that living in limbo was just too difficult to deal with and declared they would prefer that the fires came through, so at least they could then move on. I thought they were bonkers. Why would anyone wish to experience the terror of an actual bushfire?

I have given considerable thought to living in limbo and navigating the unknown. Studies have shown that many people choose to know the ending of a book or movie. They enjoy it more as they are relaxed and feel safe knowing the outcome. Others, such as I, would cover their ears and sing "la la la la la" if spoiler alerts occur. It simply doesn't make sense to me that you head straight to the end without experiencing the ride. You miss out on the actual journey. And whilst that journey may be littered with fears and trepidations, it also can be filled with joy, knowledge and fulfilment.

The COVID-19 situation tested many with the difficulties faced while living in limbo. Our lives were put on hold whilst we readjusted to a new way of existing. The frustration of restrictions, along with the risk of disease, was too stressful for some. And justifiably, anxiety and depression threatened to prevail.

I understand what it is like to live with a dark cloud lingering above your head. I know what it feels like to never quite feel free of that shadow. Often, between treatments, scans, and results, my life does get put on hold, and other times, when I feel cautiously optimistic, an anomaly on a scan or a pain will remind me that it isn't allowed. At times, it is simply tiring.

Living in limbo is pretty much permanent in my situation. However, would I choose to experience a bushfire in order to move on? Nope, not a chance.

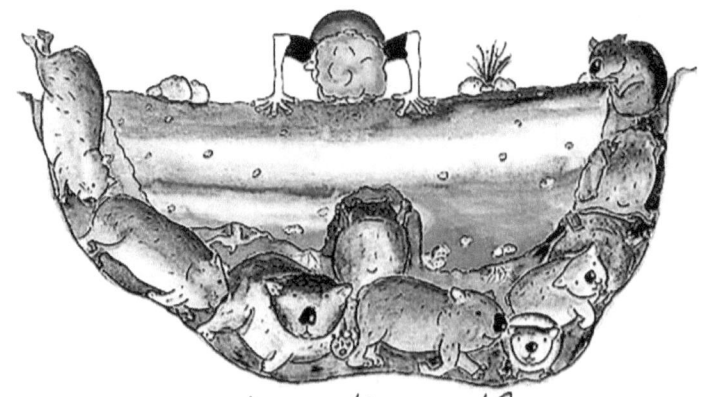

Are we there yet?

Wednesdays with Harry
CLOUDY COSMOS

Quite frankly, I am astounded I am still capable of writing anything right now as I am extremely sleep deprived. Be prepared for slurring of words, muddled metaphors and rampant ramblings.

Yesterday, Harry and I happened to be listening to Kennedy Molloy, a radio program on Triple M, when they were discussing the astronomical event about to grace our skies early this morning. Brilliant, I thought - Harry is not so keen. Unfortunately for my plans, radio host Mick Molloy explicitly argued the downside of rising at two in the morning, underdressed in the cold backyard searching for a couple of stars. The fact that Harry now had an ally in his 'stay in bed and sleep' argument only slightly diminished my enthusiasm to encourage him to agree.

Apparently, this cosmological occurrence was a combination of the sighting of the Swan Comet and the Eta Aquariids Meteor shower. An amateur astronomer from Swan Hill in Victoria discovered this comet, and it is apparently a big deal in the cosmo world. An astronomer professor from the University of Southern Queensland said, *'Comets are like cats, you try to predict what they are going to do, but they'll do their own thing anyway'*. He said it would resemble a green, fuzzy blob on the eastern horizon. Not sure that '*fuzzy green blob*' is a particular astronomical term, but goodo. The other spectacular, not to be missed, star event coinciding with the Swan Comet is the Eta Aquariids Meteor shower, which is a collection of tiny grains of dust from the tail of Halley's Comet. They hit the earth's atmosphere at about 60km per second and create lots of shooting stars. The same professor was at it again with analogies.

'They're a bit like buses – you might wait for a while, and then you might see three in a minute'. Halley's Comet was last seen in 1986 and is sighted every seventy-six years, but the dust from Halley seen this morning is likely from a fly-by thousands of years ago. Amazing.

Now, as you may imagine - ahem, Harry was fascinated with all this celestial information. He still, however, vehemently explained that under no circumstances would he leave his bed to watch such an occurrence. As he went to bed last night, the final negotiation was a little sketchy, but in my mind, he may have agreed to get up if it was worth it, and some mumbling about not being responsible for lashing out in his sleep. For my part, I knew that I didn't actually have to set the alarm, as one of our dogs has adopted the habit of needing a wee at precisely the same time every morning. She has come to realise that I am the only responsible adult in this household who will listen to her needs, and so finds me in my slumber and pesters me to be let out. Alas, the time is usually around 2.05 am.

When Mulligan nudged me awake at 2.08 am this morning, she perhaps noticed my utterings towards her were a little more gentle than usual and so, on her way out, collected her favourite ball in the hope that a game was on the cards. It does take a minute or ten to adjust to the time and the darkness. I also discovered that it takes a while to put thongs on the correct feet and for my neck muscles to behave to stare upward in a satisfactory star-gazing position. Oh, and Mick Molloy was correct - it was freezing.

So, I am teetering in the cold backyard with Mulligan licking my foot while nudging me to toss her ball, and it was then that I came to grasp the reality that there was NOT a star in the sky and definitely NO green fuzzy blob on the eastern horizon! I quickly concluded that the cat and bus analogy was utterly irrelevant; complete cloud cover was miserably hiding anything else of a cosmic nature.

Not to be completely disheartened, I decided that perhaps the clouds would pass and that 4:30 am would be a more suitable star shower time. Tottering back towards the house, I overlooked that my phone had an inbuilt torch, cursed that I couldn't see where I was going and managed to clunk my head on the one juicy lemon dangling over the path - and no, Mulligan, not playing ball!

Well, of course, there was no point waking Harry up to see a cloud, so I decided to try again at 4:30 a.m. This time, I did need to set the alarm and, of course, was horrified and confused when it actually went off. I was starting to question whether I needed to complete this particular task. However, once again, I found myself standing in the backyard, surrounded by cold air and clouds, so I finally surrendered defeat and shuffled back to bed.

Did I mention that the garbage trucks arrived very early this morning? At least Harry is awake and functioning and somewhat chuffed that he missed early morning cloud gazing…twice. I must say, though, tired as I feel, I did manage a little chuckle when I saw him run into the backyard and get clobbered by a lemon!

So there you go…

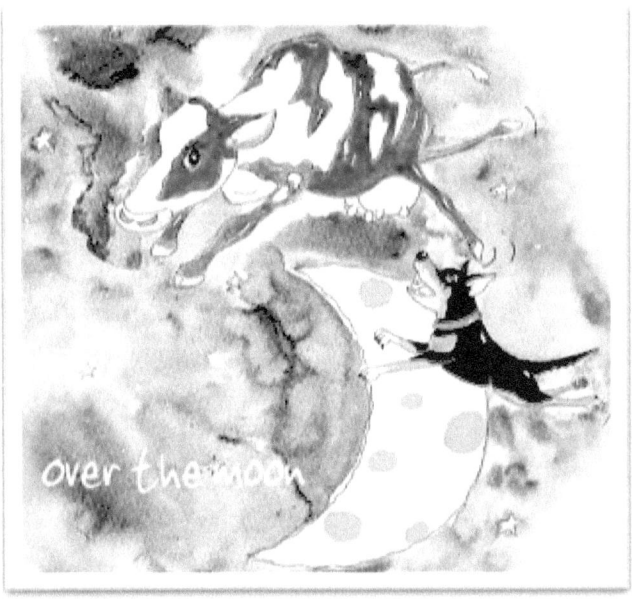

IN THE PINK
May 2014

It was now over three years since I was first diagnosed with breast cancer, and a few months since thyroid cancer had been removed. I struggled to cope with thyroxine (thyroid replacement) medication as the dose wasn't quite right. It did, however, give me insight into how chemical imbalances can really mess up your mind. The issue was that my bloodwork was telling the doctors my T4 hormone levels were acceptable, but my mental state disagreed.

Over the years, I have gained an understanding of how depression can cause serious, debilitating issues, and I am also so thankful that overall, those concerns hadn't applied to me – except for this period when the lack of a thyroid dominated my life. I suddenly felt life was hopeless and struggled to gain any positive outlook. Thoughts were weighted with doom. This struggle interfered with my day-to-day functioning, and I finally sought medical advice. The doctor told me that he had no doubt that the culmination of two cancer diagnoses would have caused such emotion and wanted to put me on depression medication. I, however, disagreed and emphasised that this had only become an issue since my thyroid had been removed and insisted that we change the thyroxine dosage. It was a bit of a battle as my blood work didn't match my own assessment. Eventually, however, I made enough noise, the medical world listened, and the dose was adjusted. Whilst this was a mentally challenging time in my life, I am so fortunate that it was temporary. It gave me a genuine appreciation for sufferers of ongoing mental health issues and how important it is for awareness, understanding, and that support is given to those affected. A cancer diagnosis quite often goes hand in hand with mental challenges. Of course, anyone affected should absolutely seek help, those close by to look out for symptoms and do whatever it takes to help.

As far as I was concerned, the chapter on thyroid cancer was pretty much closed. I would eventually see an endocrinologist to monitor any issues, but as for the cancer bit, job done. On the breast cancer front, I was feeling okay. I had finished treatment, my hair was growing back, and I only had to visit oncology every six weeks to have my portacath flushed. I began to feel that I could relax for a minute and look forward to a long and healthy future.

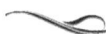

Pink is not really my colour. Not a big deal, but I prefer more earthy tones. Therefore, when I decided to join a couple of the breast cancer fundraisers, I simply had nothing to wear. The Mother's Day Walk (for some, a run) around The Tan (a 4km walking track surrounding the Botanical Gardens) in Melbourne is an annual event that sees thousands of joggers/walkers dressed in every shade of pink possible. Clearly, everyone accepted the invitation to play dress up. Sewing machines uncovered, costume shops raided, T-shirts designed, and pretty soon, The Tan became a shimmering pink wave of caterpillar movement. Every shade of pink was represented. Fuchsia stockings, salmon headscarves, flamingo tutus, bubble-gum boas, hot pink hats and rose-coloured glasses. I was walking with a few close friends. Everyone joined in and welcomed the celebration. Perhaps the simple gesture of dressing out of the ordinary promotes merriment and mirth. Laughter became the catalyst for unity, that, and of course, the cause. Underneath the smiles and sweat was the genuine understanding of why we were all there. Just like the assortment of pink hues was the various reasons to attend. For some, it was a way to contribute to raising funds; for others, it was a celebration of their breast cancer survival, and for many, it was a tribute to a loved one lost.

I'm not usually a big fan of pink-themed events, but I went all out this weekend. The night before the Mother's Day Walk, I attended the Field of Women at the Melbourne Cricket Ground. I was there with my fourteen-year-old son, Harry and his mate Ollie. It was more of a sombre occasion. One of reflection, contemplation, grief and hope.

Upon arrival, we were handed our bag of pink goodies, which included a pink raincoat and a pink filtered torch. It wasn't just about the women, as blokes can also develop breast cancer. The colour blue represented them. Thousands waited in the stands, sorting their coats in preparation for the assault onto the ground. I noticed the teams. The groups of support that surrounded and/or united with the grieving, the cancer patients and survivors. Memorial placards, tributes on T-shirts, hands-on hearts. All carefully and thoughtfully prearranged.

I was new to this type of event. Perhaps because my overall strategy was not to give cancer too much airtime, I didn't involve myself in many breast cancer occasions. And this possibly showed, as my team for the night consisted of Harry and Ollie. Both declared that the highlight, besides walking on the hallowed turf of the MCG, was illuminating their teeth by shining the pink filtered torches into their mouths. This was a good thing. They most likely saved me from becoming overly emotional, although when encircled by thousands, I couldn't ignore the overwhelming feeling of solidarity and empathy. It was poignant, spiritual and provided a cloak of compassion. However, even standing among thousands of pink-clad people, at times, I did feel quite alone.

Fifteen thousand pink raincoated, torch-carrying individuals, including Harry, Ollie, and me, formed the shape of a woman —a breast cancer symbol. I believe we were standing in the left hip region, and when the image projected onto the big screen at the 'G', well, it was a sight to behold.

So, it was a completely pink-washed weekend and gave me plenty to digest. So grateful for Harry and Ollie and their light-hearted innocence and also to those who reached out and walked The Tan.

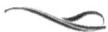

I absolutely understand the camaraderie, the unity, the comparisons and the hype. However, years later, my thoughts are more philosophical. Perhaps the humongous leap into advanced cancer has affected my views. I have grown to appreciate the complexities, variations and outcomes of cancer and realise how it all fits with me. I recognise the various colours we label cancer, but I no longer think they matter; I comprehend the comparisons but strive towards uniqueness. I realise why survival is celebrated, but I don't understand the honour it brings. I know I probably should understand, but I just don't get the whole 'survivor' network surrounding cancer. Of course, I know the use of the word. It is entirely appropriate to say you are a cancer survivor. I understand how relief would be an overwhelming emotion if you are fortunate to get the all-clear. I imagine the celebrations would be justified; your zest for life would be reinstated when your future is offered precious time and liberty. I get all that. You have survived something horrendous, and indeed, it is something to be proud of, but I don't particularly understand the need to wear it like a badge of honour, proudly displaying your cancer-fighting achievements. '*I am a cancer survivor*' is plastered on t-shirts with dedicated chest-puffing and prominence. Perhaps it is showcased to promote hope and inspire others? That makes sense, but could it also be that it simply represents the fact that you have gone through a really crappy and scary time, and you are proud that you live to tell the tale? And that is certainly worth noting, but what makes someone survive when others don't? I wonder if a cancer survivor means that you had treatable cancer that wouldn't end your life. You may have experienced an enormous scare and had to endure gruelling and savage treatment with hideous side effects that may be temporary, permanent or lingering. But what makes one person actually survive over someone who doesn't? Is it their will to live, their positivity, their alternative therapies, their prayer, their mental strength, their wishes or their hopes? Or is it simply that no one dies of 'curable' cancer? I know, using that 'curable' word again.

If we view cancer survivors as a success, does that mean that those who have died or have incurable cancer are failures? If the benchmark of being part of the 'survivors' club means that you get to live without cancer, then those who are perpetually attached to treatment are not welcome. You stand up and proudly declare that you went into battle with a beast, and you won. Perhaps the more apt slogan of being a 'cancer survivor' should be '*I survived cancer treatment*'. Because maybe that is what this is about. You were mentally and physically challenged by health. You may have had surgery, radiotherapy and chemo, and you may have felt incredible fear, and maybe you still do feel fear and live in limbo. You may have been positive and inspirational throughout. You may have discovered a strength you didn't know existed. You may have a more grateful and appreciative outlook and have sorted out what is important to you. But ultimately, that struggle, and the changes are about a diagnosis and treatment. The reality is that you have survived something treatable. You were put into a fearful state of mind because of how we all think of cancer. I get it. I felt the same.

Everything changes, however, when you are told your life will end because of cancer, and you will not be a survivor.

I have lived many years since first being diagnosed with stage three breast cancer, and now over a decade since being labelled terminal. Some may classify me as a survivor. I don't class myself as anything to do with cancer. I had treatment, I still have treatment, and I find a way to cope with the reminders that I am in stage four.

Because here is another question - if we object to being defined by cancer, then why is being defined as a 'cancer survivor' any different? Ultimately, we are still letting cancer present as something prominent and powerful.

I had a look at the various 'cancer survivor' groups, and here is a quote from one of them. '*Cancer in all stages is traumatic to a person receiving that diagnosis. Cancer of any kind is petrifying to have – because IT'S CANCER.*' Of course, this is an acceptable statement, but it is also the reason why we are all scared out of our wits at the very mention of a cancer diagnosis. Isn't it about time we recognised cancer's various stages and prognosis, and try to quieten the fear?

I am genuinely not underestimating anyone's own cancer experience, but I have witnessed cancer become more than a disease of the body so many times. Its destruction and intrusion into the mind can be challenging to overcome. All I can truly do is attempt to deal with the facts, try to look after my mental wellbeing, be mindful, accountable and honest.

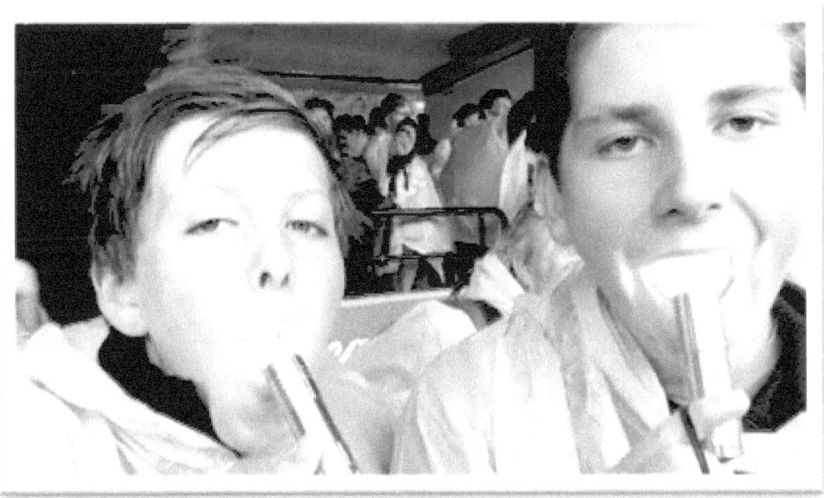

Wednesdays with Harry
ORGANISING CHAOS

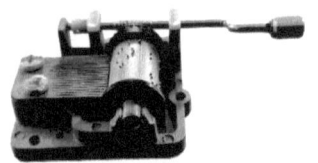

Yesterday was a planned outage here in Warburton. I am starting to believe this book is simply a diary of local power outages. Fortunately for Harry, he had his phone and laptop humming on long-life batteries and hooked up to my hotspot and therefore, his day was seemingly unaffected. On the other hand, I favour a desktop computer to work from and am far too old and stubborn to try and utilise my phone as a replacement. As my computer was out of action, I decided to spend the day cleaning out cupboards and drawers in my office. I guess I could have chosen to tidy the Tupperware cupboard, but that task requires one to have at least six weeks of mental and physical preparation. There is perhaps a TAFE course on Structural and Organisational Engineering that one should seriously consider before undertaking such a mission.

So, I began with what I assumed would be the least difficult, and that was my desk drawer. I soon discovered that whilst the size of the drawer appeared regular, it proved to be quite the bottomless pit. Years of squirrelling away the most useless bits of junk resulted in me questioning the need for any of it and so reached for a big black garbage bag. I did pause when I spied among the multiple tattered business cards, old ink cartridges, and three bottles of crusty white-out correction fluid, a small wind-up musical thingy. I plucked it out, gave it a twirl and the metal tongs clipped onto the pimpled cylinder to the melodic tune of '*Imagine*'. After playing with my new, not so new, toy for a while, I decided I had better be more thorough in checking for any other keepsakes. You will be pleased to know that whilst I tossed plenty of inkless pens, bent paperclips, shopping lists, dried glue sticks, and a 2005 take away menu from Woks of Fire, I did manage to rescue a fragrant sachet, an *It's a Girl* greeting card and tickets to see Neil Diamond from his cancelled tour.

No such excitement was repeated when I tackled the shelves and the cupboard. Sure, it's handy to know that I have enough sticky tape to last until 2030 and that when storing craft glue, it's wise to put a lid on and store upright. I did, however, come across a couple of old High School yearbooks that instantly transported me back to a simpler time, and when life was relatively harmonious. Whilst it is all relative, it is quite likely that if you considered anxiety was whether you arrived home, after travelling on the school bus, with your Home Economics black forest cherry cake intact or not, then you really had few concerns.

Having a gander at these yearbooks, the first glaringly obvious question I needed to ask was, why did our school call them Salamander? And why didn't I think that was an odd choice of title when I was actually at school? Having a yearbook named after a somewhat unattractive amphibian, newt-type creature, is indeed a mystery. Some of their features include blunt snouts, short limbs that project at right angles to their bodies, and the presence of a tail. Perhaps an apt description of many students on sports days?

It was fascinating to dive back in time, and it was even worth the cringy feeling when faced with what I looked like. The 70's fashion and hairstyles are perhaps the true answer to the Salamander question.

Well, the cupboards are tidy, the shelves are dust-free, and my drawers are now hungry for new junk!

Postscript: I have since discovered the reason our yearbook was named Salamander. It seems that they represent immortality and rebirth, but also can resist fire due to the 'milky substance' produced by their skin. Apparently, our school was also able to withstand an arson attempt. So there you go...

THOUGHTS FROM CLOSE BY

It's all very well acknowledging the impact of cancer from my perspective, but its tentacles reach beyond just me. I thought it would be a significant inclusion to also peer in from another viewpoint. I have asked friends and family if they wanted to contribute. (Family is on page 189) My idea was that it is simply a collection of thoughts and emotions about how or if cancer had affected them. I am touched, but perhaps it has eventuated to be not so much about them and their own lives, but as a tribute to myself. To avoid mushy, embarrassing praise and homage, please feel free to skip this bit.

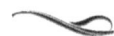

When my best friend told me she had been diagnosed with cancer, I was devastated. I felt sad, hopeless, and frustrated that my beautiful friend had been dealt such a terrible hand. Since Jo's diagnosis, we have shared many ups and downs, and she never ceases to amaze me with her positive attitude towards her illness and her ability to get straight back up after being knocked down. I believe Jo makes me see her cancer differently than I felt the first time when I learnt of her diagnosis. She lives her life and doesn't let cancer define who she is. Jo is always interested in helping others, and she is one of the most inspirational women I have ever met. I am so honoured to call you my friend, Jo. Love Penny xxxx

I remember when Jo told me of her first diagnosis, and I still have the scribble on a pink post-it note in my bottom drawer with some keywords.
- Stage 3 aggressive
- Not a hormonal cancer
- 23 lymph nodes removed
- Starting treatment for 18 months
- 2 - 3% get this type of breast cancer

And that was only what I had scribbled, as there was more to it.

I was sitting on the side of my bed looking out over the front driveway and garden, and with tears streaming down my face, thinking FARKKKKKK. How can this be? What can I do to help, and then you realise you can't do anything except to be on deck to chat or listen. My immediate thoughts went to Harry.

And so, the journey began. I have often asked how on earth she has got through this with all the associated health issues over the years and continued to write, publish, create, build a business, and have so much energy. But that's who she is, an absolute go-getter who is determined to live her life her way and not let this disease win. And with the love of her family & friends, she has succeeded.
Leanne

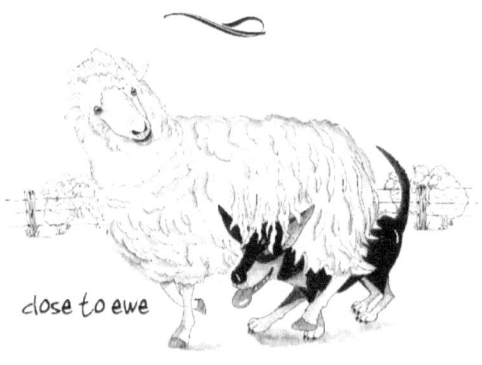

I hate that you have to live with your diagnosis every day. I hate what you have been through to survive and what your body and mind have to endure. I hate that you have had to envision a life for Harry without you. Your thoughtfulness and generosity haven't diminished while undergoing lifesaving treatment, which has robbed you of so many things. You are beautiful, generous, and creative and don't deserve this, which upsets me the most. I can't believe how you're always there for me, and I hope you feel I am here for you too. My issues are nothing compared to yours. I am crying while writing this. You are so loved. Annette.

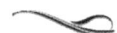

*W*hen Jo asked me to contribute to Chasing Normal, I was a bit daunted because it meant thinking about my feelings and for me, it's been a weird old decade of everything but 'normal' (does normal even exist?) on so many levels, including having a dear friend facing complex health issues. I admit that I am prone to burying my head in the sand and not thinking much beyond getting through the next day.

I remember very clearly the day that we got news of Jo's breast cancer diagnosis because she didn't want to talk – and that's a rare thing for the Jo I know, so I knew it wasn't a good sign. Everything seemed to move very quickly from diagnosis to mastectomy to chemo and radiation therapy. Throughout it all, there have been very few times that Jo has let the enormity of the situation knock her fierce determination not to be defined by her cancer. I recall a conversation about joining support groups, but Jo believed that by spending hours *talking or grieving something that has no rhyme or reason or sense of fairness, you're effectively giving power to the disease and letting it control you. I often wondered if this attitude has helped her stay well, despite all the additional and ongoing health complications (and other cancers) she's dealing with.*

We have laughed over prosthetics and wigs, and debated plant-based diets, alternative therapies and the unpredictability of how humans react to cancer. Some people can't deal, don't know what to say, and avoid any conversation.

Last year, I wrote an article (in my professional capacity) about a project Jo was working on, and it encouraged me to think about how she has faced her unique (and complex) cancer experience. I've extracted a paragraph from the piece that sums up the way I've seen Jo approach everything:

'Jo has been a good friend of mine for 13 years now. She's a positive person who doesn't like to focus on herself [and is] fuelled [by] her desire to help others. Over the years, I have witnessed her strength and courage dealing with hours of surgeries and ongoing treatment, sometimes with horrid side effects. Some days she accepts that she feels rotten; not much will happen on either a domestic or professional level - she just needs to get through the day - but most days, she just carries on and refuses to let cancer define her life. Jo has learned to listen to her body and is surrounded by family who are happy to help...but she still works hard. She is the most productive person I have ever met and, despite her health challenges, has continued to write and create prolifically over the last few years.'

I also spoke about Jo's eternally positive outlook, but also acknowledged the whole spectrum of emotions that come from facing our own mortality. Her own experience has given her great empathy for others, whilst being super-aware that everyone's experience is completely unique. Focusing outward and 'chasing normal' have been so important for her.

It's an unbearable thought to think about losing a friend. We don't talk about it often, but I know that being given a 'timeline' for her cancer and being told it is terminal has been frustrating because, while she prefers to focus on getting on with life, it's hard not to wonder about the accuracy of the medical prognosis. It's been a burden for her to have those words in the back of her mind. We both agree that this is sometimes unhelpful – especially for someone like Jo, whose complex situation has provided a unique challenge for the health system and their prognosis inaccurate and pointless. A less determined and curious person may not have questioned some of the advice she's received; her gut feeling to go against initial diagnoses has served her well.

Neither of us knows what the years ahead hold, but by recognising what is and what is not within our control and accepting that there will no doubt be some rough with the smooth, we will face each day as it comes. We all want to be there for Jo. I have no doubt that she will face life's smoother bits in exactly the same no-nonsense way that she always has. I hope she knows that I'll still be there on the rough days. Jo's cancer is sometimes a reminder of life's unexpected and unpredictable nature and how we take so much for granted. She has made me appreciate the little things. Pip

Wednesdays with Harry
MOUNTAIN ASH

Finally, we completed an activity together, albeit a short one, but an activity no less.

As I sit writing this, the sun is bursting through the office window, seemingly virtuous but in fact tainted with complete indifference to the fact that only one hour earlier, it had gone missing, abandoned us and was replaced by rain. Perhaps lousy timing on our behalf, or maybe it was meant to be, for what more appropriate weather to visit a rain forest than when it is raining?

Ten minutes up the mountain from home is Cement Creek, and a walk in the tree canopy and forest floor. Cement Creek. Not the most romantic name for a beautiful, pristine waterway; however, it is named after the conglomerate rock formations. The magnificent abundance of nature was immediately highlighted by glimpsing an elusive lyrebird dart across the road before disappearing into the forest. It was too quick for the camera, but as it scurried away, it left a glorious impression with its ostentatious and elaborate feathered tail.

The view from the canopy walk is magical, and you are encircled and humbled by the magnificent Mountain Ash. Testing my short, stubby neck in this unnatural position was either going to enable me to appreciate the impressive height and command of these trees or indeed cause vertigo and a complete blackout!

Fortunately, I lived to tell the tale and continued on our soggy but satisfying walk. As it was raining, we were wearing what should be considered waterproof attire. Anyone reading any past posts would realise that the coat I continue to wear in dodgy weather, contrary to appearance, is, in fact, not at all waterproof, and yes, I need to acquire a more appropriate coat. Harry, of course, was sporting a brand-name coat and was indignant at the idea that it was anything less than waterproof.

The next stage of this walk was to venture down to the forest floor. It always seems innocuous to mention that you are venturing 'down' - until, of course, you must venture 'up'. More of that in a moment.

On the way, the luminous, shimmering foliage of ferns lines the path. I push aside the thought that blood-sucking leeches may be lying in wait and try to outsmart my camera's warning that I need to defog my lens. In doing so, I discovered that I have camera options that I had previously been ignorant of. Harry is absolutely no help when it comes to explaining the technology. He obstinately believes that it is not his responsibility to assist and instruct on issues that I can work out myself. I reminded him that he was considering changing his degree to become a teacher, which, by definition, is a career in instruction. His silence was either a protest or a sign of defeat, but either way, I did figure it out myself.

I was contently snapping away at the moss and the fungi until Harry broke his silence to suggest that we move quicker. It then became apparent that the 'up' was about to begin.

I have noticed lately that my left hip is a little sore, and as the 'up' involved countless steps, my pace was seriously compromised - well, that and the fact that I am incredibly unfit. Harry, of course, is a fitness freak and proceeded to leave me with the leeches and sprinted to the top. By the time I reached the car park, I had questioned my will to live and then wondered if a defibrillator could be located. Harry was waiting, not at all patiently, and was exasperated at the size of the steps I was taking.

'You know, Mum, if you took longer strides, you would get places faster, ' Harry exclaimed.

Yes, Harry, but I'm not sure I would be alive to tell the tale. So there you go...

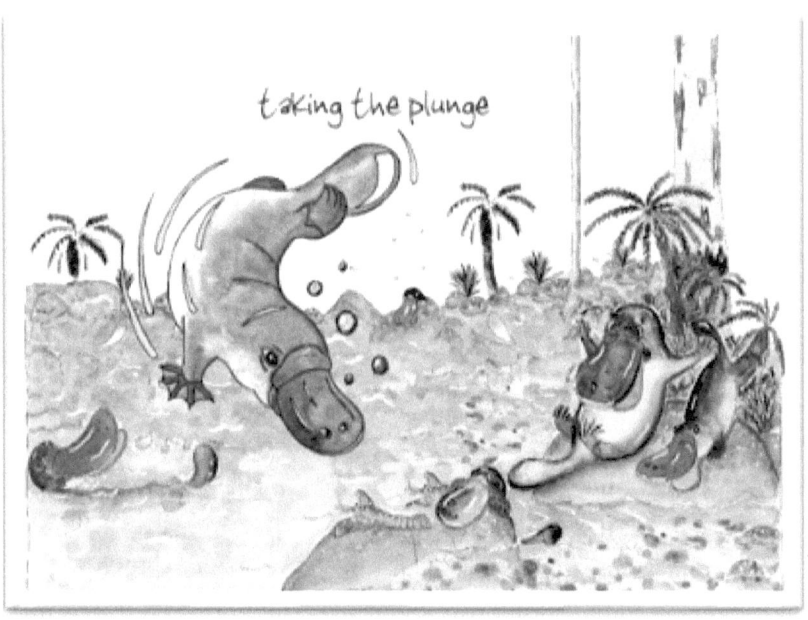

METASTATIC MONDAY
JUNE 15th, 2015

It is incredibly difficult to describe the wave of emotion that comes when you are informed, that according to all medical knowledge and statistics, your cancer is no longer curable, and you have only a few more years to live. I had always been told it was likely to return, but I still wasn't prepared for the overwhelming and desperate magnitude of disbelief. The initial fear assaults your mind to the point where numbness again is the only retreat. I look back to when first diagnosed and realise that I knew nothing. Whatever I felt then was insignificant to the weight of grief that enveloped me now.

I still clearly remember the appointment at the Breast Clinic with the Oncologist. An anomaly in my lung had been detected on a routine scan and required further investigation. Another scan was completed, and a follow-up appointment was scheduled for Monday, June 15th. When I arrived, it was another long wait. Before the new building was built, the Breast Clinic took up residence in an old house. The waiting room was small and often overcrowded. I usually chose to sit on one of the two benches placed on the outside verandah. It meant my time waiting was spent adjacent to reality. It was my attempt to avoid the escalating anxiety that I often felt in the cancer clinic waiting room, and escaping outside afforded me a small distance from the reason I was there.

On that particular day, however, I knew I had a reason for concern.

Whilst waiting, my mind kept drifting back to a class I had attended years ago when lymphedema was first diagnosed. My lymph nodes had been removed from my right armpit area, and I had contracted lymphedema. Put simply, it is an incurable condition caused by a blocked lymphatic system. The result is constant swelling of my arm. I need to be careful, as your lymphatic system is part of your immune system, so infections can be an issue.

There were about twenty attendees at this particular class, and it mainly consisted of cancer patients who had lymph nodes removed, like me. I observed that many participants were currently in treatment, as the usual scarves and hats advertised the tell-tale insignia of chemotherapy. One woman who was wearing a pink woollen beanie had the look of someone quite ill. When an opportunity came for her to speak, she explained that her cancer was stage four and advanced. She stated that there would never again be a time when she wouldn't be in treatment, nor would she ever have hair again. Her desperate look of despair demanded heartfelt sympathy and sorrow. The empathy directed towards her was palpable, and I wanted to reach out and steal away her fears. I suspected she knew her fate was sealed. And then, skirting those emotions was the self-centred thought that you were thankful it wasn't you.

Waiting on the verandah, reliving that lymphedema class, I came to the very likely realisation that that could now be me.

Finally, I was called in, and my oncologist inquired if anyone was with me today. As it wasn't usual that anyone would accompany me, I knew right then I was in for bad news. She gently explained that cancer had now spread to my lungs, which meant stage four, metastatic and incurable.

A pinball of anguish ricocheted in my mind, pinging fear and despair about in random and erratic directions. The thud of desolation was deafening.

Without really thinking whether I actually wanted to hear the reply, I went ahead and asked the question. How long? She assured me that as the nodules were small, I still had time. She could only refer to statistics, which could mean three to four years. She told me the best option was to go back on chemo. My thoughts were pretty well mush by that point. I just wanted to get out of there. I explained that I really couldn't face lining up and organising more appointments. Of course, she would handle that, and she guided me out without interruption.

My car was parked just around the corner, and as I approached, I saw my sister. She had thought to come and check on me. I managed to unlock the car and sat in the passenger seat, overcome with nausea. Gai quickly realised that the news wasn't good, and nothing would help alleviate the emotion and pain. We drove to our parents' home and were joined by the rest of the family. An ocean of tears was shed. Again, I realised this was not just about me; it was also about all who were close and, most of all, Harry.

Honestly, how do I tell my child that it was unlikely I would be here for him in the future? The conversation was brief. I did not elaborate on explaining the worst. He did become emotional, but his reliance and trust in me being okay was strong. It really didn't matter if Harry's coping system was to exist in denial or not.

So many emotions and thoughts shifted on that day in June 2015. All the stuff that I thought was important just wasn't. I came to realise the difference between earlier-stage cancers and advanced cancers is vast. You think you know what cancer is all about in the early days, but you simply don't.

The impact when you are given a shortened life expectancy is – well, I really have few words.

flipping out

Wednesdays with Harry
SNOW REGRETS

For whatever reason, Harry has a week off from University. I imagine there is a valid reason for such a break; however, it is unlikely that information will become known to me. The emphasis on completing assignments, essays, quizzes and any other educational-related obligation was moderately noted. It did become apparent that these academic commitments would be juggled with the more tempting desire to complete gym workouts, twenty-kilometre runs, and securing a front-row seat to watch the Ashes cricket test match on the telly. I suggested to Harry that he should indeed be able to find the time to do something together today. The expectation that he would declare it impossible was quickly quashed as he enthusiastically suggested that we should journey up the hill and go to the snow. He may possibly have noticed that my keenness did not come close to matching his, and this, I might add, cemented his determination for such an outing. I sensed this was payback for all the museums and galleries he agreed to partake in. So, I had little choice but to go along with the plan and gear up for the snow.

Living in Warburton means that we are at the base of Mount Donna Buang, and so a fifteen-minute drive can see us up the top and instantly frolicking in the snow. Yes, that sounds like fun and attracts many locals and tourists to also frolic. So, you may be wondering why I seem a tad hesitant. Well, firstly, it is cold. Secondly, I don't have a warm waterproof coat. Thirdly, it is cold. Fourthly, it was raining, and did I mention that it was cold? I did, however, know that we own ski gloves, snow boots and a toboggan, but I just needed to recall where they were. These items fall under the 'need to keep but don't often use' category and are stored in areas with other such items. When the mystery is finally solved, you take note in discovering that your search also uncovered NYE party hats, a mouldy air mattress and the game of Kerplunk. Anyway, I quickly adopted a less woosy attitude and faith that at least my hands and feet would be warm.

Throughout our Wednesday's activities, you may have noticed that Harry's understanding of wearing appropriate clothes to match the weather conditions has often been questionable. Today, this mindset continued. I reminded him that he did own an actual ski jacket, pants, gloves and snow boots. He declared that it wasn't too cold and that he had a coat in the car. As my precautions were clearly being ignored, I felt it necessary to reiterate my suggestion that an actual ski jacket, designed specifically for venturing into cold and wet snow, would be more suitable. He reiterated to me that he would be fine.

Well, of course, he wasn't. On exiting the car near the peak of the mountain, Harry was a little apprehensive that his new Nike runners and non-waterproof puffy jacket might not be up for the task. Fortunately, Harry's mum had the foresight to throw in his snow boots and gloves. The question then arises whether he was more annoyed that the weather was not as he expected, or the undeniable irritation that he should have taken his mother's advice. I suspect a little of both.

Quickly setting aside clothing issues, we strode to the summit. I had the idea to create a snowman, and Harry had the plan to destroy. The remains of several lifeless abandoned snowmen, plus a random tourist's picnic hamper, were the subject of friendly fire and violent abuse as snowballs were hurled in their direction.

Fortunately, reprieve came as the toboggan run beckoned. The usual maverick approach of snow surfing the hill was put into action, as tumbles, somersaults, and full-body slides managed to wipe out and face-plant the snow. This, of course, tested the non-waterproof puffy jacket's snow playability, and Harry finally concluded that a ski jacket may have been appropriate, as he was now cold and wet.

As my own coat had reached waterlogged capacity quite some time ago, I had no issue calling it quits - and did I mention that it was cold?

So there you go…

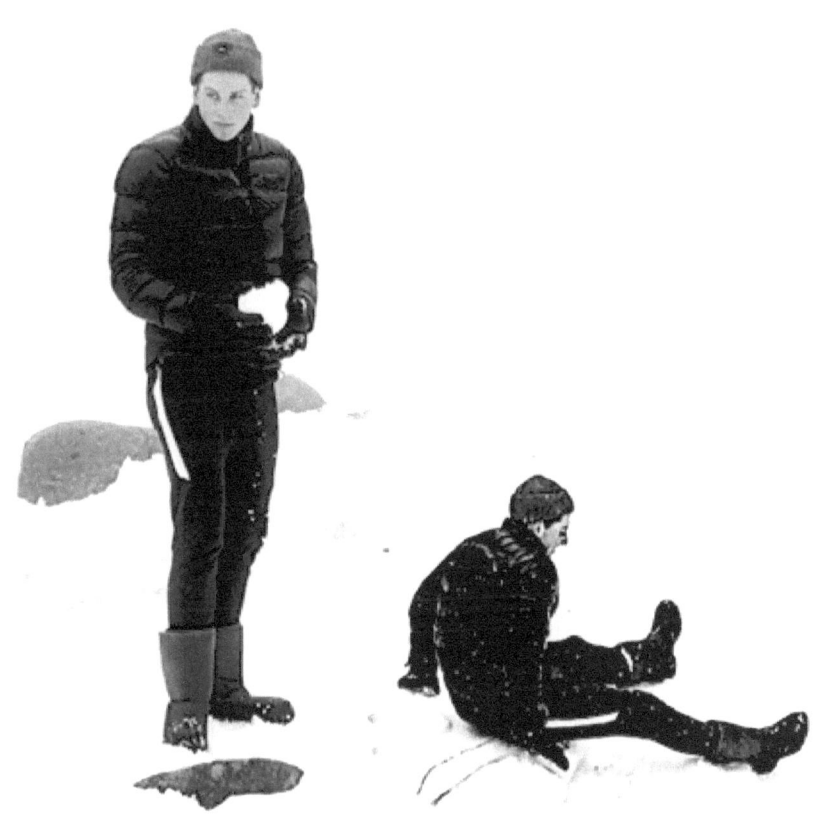

SIDEWAY EFFECTS

With a week to spare before chemotherapy dominated my life again, I packed a bag and convinced Harry that a quick road trip to the north of Victoria would be ideal. I love road trips. It provides the perfect opportunity to sing along to '80s music, munch on snacks whilst driving untroubled and carefree. Harry is rarely keen, but on this occasion, with only a whimper of dissent, he agreed to tag along. Four days of blissful, indulgent freedom ensued. Thoughts of cancer and chemo diminished as we ventured to Beechworth, Rutherglen and Echuca.

Safe to say that I wasn't looking forward to rocking up to begin chemotherapy for a second time. I had been there before, and so no part of ignorance would save me from knowing. The actual details of what is required to get through chemo is perhaps individual and dependent on the particular drugs you are administered. Suffice it to say, for me, it was far from a walk in the park. The second time around, I was instantly transported back to 2011 as I felt the toxins entering my body. Polluted. Contaminated. Physically, I hadn't truly recovered from the first time, so I didn't hold much hope for it becoming easier. It was also getting harder to believe that chemo was the answer, as cancer had indeed returned. But then again, this time was never going to be curative. This time was about prolonging life. As I wasn't brave or educated enough to walk an alternative route, I had no option but to accept what I felt had to be.

After four months of three-weekly treatments, it was decided that the peripheral neuropathy that was affecting my hands and feet was getting out of control.

Neuropathy is one of the more debilitating effects of treatment. It simply means that nerve damage has occurred in my fingers and toes. It creates a constant pins-and-needles type sensation along with aches and pains. It also means my fine motor skills are pretty much crap. The frustration from dexterity deficiencies is daily.

Chemo was therefore stopped and replaced by a targeted treatment. Along with the change in treatment, CT and bone scans were taken. They initially came back clear. Reprieve. Relief. You would think 'rejoice' would also be nestled in there, but somehow that felt like I was tempting fate. Low-key relief was as good as it gets. It now becomes a constant waiting game between three monthly scans. Future scans would show nodules come and go. Some small, some larger. My case has been, and continues to be, discussed among various doctors to determine the mystery. And in between, we wait. Every scan taken has been added to the jigsaw created to establish my own cancer picture, and in the meantime, treatment and side effects continue.

When I talk about the side effects of cancer, I am usually acknowledging the crappiness of treatment. However, the mental side effects can have their own complete category.

Not sure if vanity counts as a side effect, but on occasion, my one-breasted, patchy hair and scarred aging body can thwart my usual pragmatic attitude. Now, don't let my photo on the first page fool you. Behind the blurry paintbrush filter lies hundreds of telltale signs of years of toxic chemicals, stress and aging. Those who believe wrinkles create character and should be proudly worn to indicate a life well-lived, may be confusing my facial creases as laugh lines, and from spending the last decade sunning myself on the Costa del Sol!

Of course, I realise that vanity in the world of cancer seems incredibly trivial and unimportant. Even mentioning this is subjecting my superficiality to being exposed and inviting judgemental opinions. Because clearly, when diagnosed with a terminal disease, concern about looks is seen as shallow and a completely egotistical waste of energy. On the surface, it is easy to assume that, like many women my age, I just don't wish to see my face sliding south. Underneath, it is more than that. It is beyond vanity. It is a pent-up frustration of feeling cheated that any resemblance of youth has been stripped away and replaced by toxins and stress from years of treatment and concern.

Our looks are a statement of time. Does what I look like matter to anyone else? No. Not a debate, just how I feel.

Having said that, in my defence, I don't believe I have spent too many hours wallowing in vanity over the years. Well, except for that time back in my late teens...

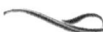

In my youth, I played field hockey, and in 1979 our team reached the grand final. Hockey was played in the winter months, which ensured my legs, protruding from a very short hockey skirt, were blindingly white. The night before the match, in a moment of complete insanity, I decided that Marching Girl Tan was the remedy. You need to remember that this was back when fake tan was a relatively new product, and there were very few options available. Unbeknownst to me at the time, it came with the guarantee of creating a streaky orange mess, along with an overwhelming stench.

Having not used this product previously, I felt confident that my quest to look fit and sun-kissed would definitely be achieved.

I was horrified when I woke to discover that my legs were not only incandescently tangerine, but they also secreted a pungent, musky pong. My attempts to scrub it off seemed only to result in a more permanent application. With no time to seek further advice or solution, I put on my uniform, added tracky daks and joined the team.

The match was about to start, and my edginess had little to do with playing a grand final and more to do with the fact that my tracksuit had to come off. Needless to say, my legs were noticed.

My horror continued when, during the match, I began to observe that my socks were changing colour. Apparently, Marching Girl Tan, mixed with sporty sweat, created a runoff effect. Unfortunately, this was also highlighted when I needed physical therapy attention when a leg cramp crippled my run in the game's later stages. I could not have been more mortified, not only when the first-aid trainer bloke had to rub my stinky tangelo legs, but when he finally realised why his hands were stained and tinted orange!

Fortunately, we won the premiership, which, of course, was fabulous and created a worthwhile and sizable diversion from my embarrassment. It's safe to say that I have not used fake tan since, and vanity has taken quite a back seat.

But back to my current wrinkly groan…regardless of my rabbiting on about looks, of course, I am thankful I am still here, irrespective of the side effects. There is an overriding expectation, a feeling that others expect you never to feel anything less. I don't feel I am allowed to complain about treatment, or lymphedema or peripheral neuropathy, or having one breast or hair issues and definitely not about wrinkles because, well, firstly, so many others have crappier problems than me, AND I need to be eternally grateful that I am alive. I get it. I am lucky to look old or reach a certain age or even feel pain because so many others in my situation haven't had that privilege.

Most of the time, my cancer perspective is one of gratitude, acceptance, and appreciation. But some days it isn't.

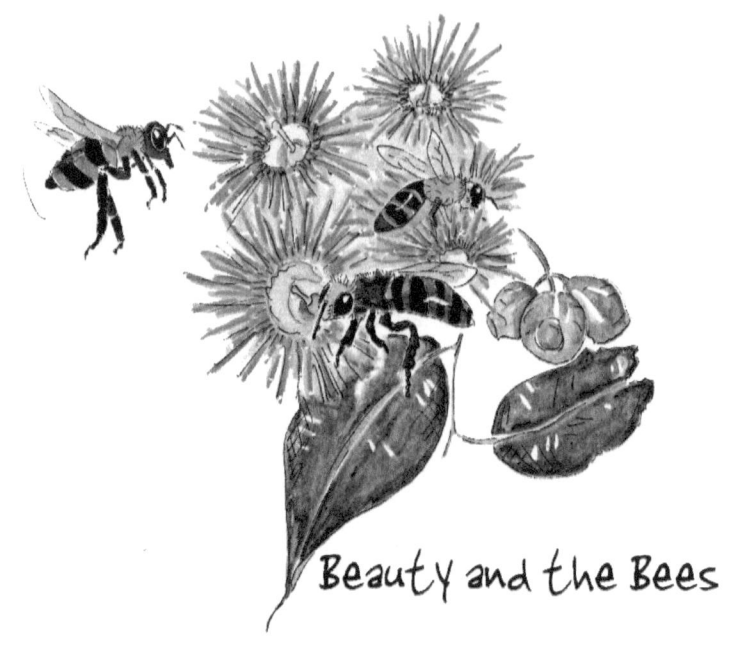
Beauty and the Bees

Wednesdays with Harry
GREAT OCEAN ROAD

Between the start of a new University year for Harry and scooting around to several appointments myself, we found ourselves with four days on which we were both keen to have a mini holiday.

I suggested various Victorian locations whilst Harry began to research fares to Noosa. After putting the kibosh on that idea and convincing him (not really) that Lorne was the Noosa of the south, we packed our bags and headed off down the Great Ocean Road.

It wasn't long before the usual tug of war began in selecting a radio station. As the steering wheel houses a button that controls radio options, I believe choice and power belong to the driver. So, with Don McLean and me warbling out all thirty-four verses of American Pie, our journey began. I suspect that whilst Harry appeared somewhat impassive, he secretly admired the fact that I knew ALL the words. Ahh, yes, the glimpses of confusion when your child occasionally realises that you actually had a life before they came to exist. And what a life it was!

Eventually, the battle over radio rights was inconsequential as all stored stations screamed static ruckus until they were deemed kaput. Finally, we happened upon a local radio station, and so, with no other option, we settled on K-Rock – Home of the Hits.

There are likely those reading this who are screaming with frustration and totally bewildered by our lack of foresight in not plugging in a phone and using music playlists. I blame Harry for such oversight, and so, finally, on day two, when K-Rock - Home of the Hits started to flounder, the light bulb moment occurred. Hello! An extraordinary plethora of musical choices was now discovered.

Now, what is not to love about Lorne? Brilliant destination and we had accommodation just moments away from the sea. As soon as my toes touched the sand, I melted into a more relaxed version of myself. Perhaps memories of carefree summers spent holidaying at the beach triggers an instant calm…that is, of course, unless the heat becomes an issue. Every redhead knows that a painful attack of sunburn is just moments away when playing with solar power. We travel with a collection of SPF 50+ sunscreen lotions, multiple arrays of wide-brimmed headwear and cover our limbs in anti-sun material. Our natural ability to seek out a canopy is first-rate, and we will physically threaten to harm others who steal our shade. Fortunately for all concerned, the weather in Lorne was just right.

Erskine Falls offered a remarkable natural setting, along with a real test of my lung capacity. Always be cautious of vertical descents that require a return. Passing many fellow tourists huffing their way up should have been fair warning that this body would be pushed to the limit. Of course, fitness freak Harry was totally unsympathetic with my heaving issues, whilst I questioned the date of our ambulance subscription.

So, it is obviously ridiculous to venture along the Great Ocean Road without agreeing to be blown away by photographing the Twelve Apostles and Loch Ard Gorge. This part of the trip is when you play tag with fellow tourists, some of whom you recognised from Erskine Falls. Every sightseeing bay you meet and politely nod in recognition. The leather-jacket-wearing, seventy-five-year-old Motley Crew loving couple who had overindulged in black hair dye; the family trying to restrain their children from falling off the cliff; the youthful females attempting to control their hair extensions, and the middle-aged couple trying to find a toilet.

We read the relevant, informative signs and noted the tragic outcomes along the Shipwreck Coast. One of the repeated warnings clearly explains that there are fragile cliffs and venomous snakes.

Feeling quite blasé about both issues was my downfall. Managed to negotiate the fragile cliffs but failed to notice, until almost stepping upon, a couple of snakes sunning themselves on a path. Most likely, they were entirely oblivious to my utter terror and overreaction; however, I didn't stick around long enough to ever know.

Definitely not a fan of reptiles of a slithery nature, but finally, Harry was able to witness me moving with the swiftness of speed he approved.

Well, four days is not a particularly long holiday, but we both really enjoyed the break.

So there you go…

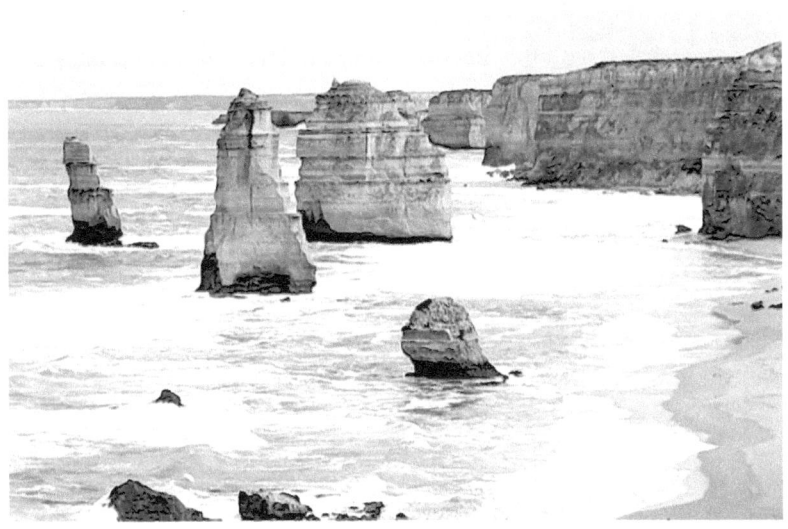

R.I.P. REBECCA WILSON

October 7th, 2016

Today I woke to the news that Rebecca Wilson had passed away. It was breast cancer, and she was fifty-four years old. I didn't know Rebecca personally; however, I felt incredibly saddened and quite overwhelmed with grief. I remember her as the feisty yet humorous sports journalist and a regular panellist on the television program The Fat – a light-hearted sports show hosted by Tony Squires. More recently, I had listened to her radio commentary. I liked her style. She had moxie. According to the reports, she kept the news about her breast cancer private from many friends and family members in order to limit their suffering.

The glaringly obvious comparison that I have metastatic breast cancer, coupled with the fact that I will be fifty-four next month, has sent me spinning into a whirlwind of thoughts, questions, feelings and emotions. My usually logical, rational, common-sense mind has been knocked off-kilter. I do realise that we are all individuals, and Rebecca's cancer was also individual, so why do I feel compelled to write what I think when her story is not mine? I recall that this response has happened before, and I wonder if it's the same for others in this situation.

Do we put ourselves in another's story to try and make sense of our own?

I think about the fact that she kept the diagnosis private. I understand the need to protect those around you from suffering. There is a resilient and defiant strength in doing so. I question my openness about my own diagnosis and wonder if I should have kept it quiet. I think, however, that whether you share your diagnosis or not, having cancer creates a very lonely place. No one else can truly understand what you feel. I can share my thoughts, hoping that they may offer insight or relate to those also going through it, but the reality is that only you know the depth of your own emotions. Facing your mortality is solitary.

Just as I was in the middle of writing this, I received a phone call from a very dear friend. She rang just to say hi, but knew that my reaction to Rebecca's passing may have affected me. If she hadn't been aware of my situation, she wouldn't have known to reach out and call. So yes, having cancer is lonely, but knowing that others are empathetic and are standing by your side on these kinds of days is such a blessing and gives me strength.

The reality of cancer and its potential outcome was very present with me today. But I hold on very tightly to the thought that I am my own story. It is a day to grieve for Rebecca's story, and throughout the day, I have discovered it is also a day for me to feel grateful.

The comparison is unnecessary because the significant difference that is so abundantly clear is that I am still here.

Rest in peace, Rebecca Wilson.

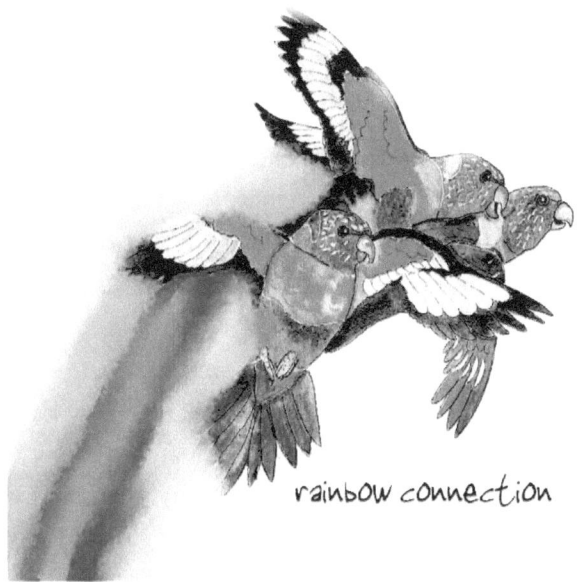

rainbow connection

Wednesdays with Harry
TRIPLE ANTARTIC BLAST

Not quite sure why I chose today to try and remedy my limited eyelash situation. I found a couple of falsies in the back of the drawer and decided to take aim at the scared, stubbly lashes that remained. For those younger than fifty, the sagging, wrinkly skin situation that occupies the top of my eyelids may not be an evident frustration for false eyelash application. In addition, failing eyesight thwarts placement accuracy, leaving lashes protruding, lopsided and askew. In retrospect, I may have applied a little too much glue, as I spent the next five hours unable to blink.

Triple Antarctic Blast – headlined the news this morning. Possibly, it doesn't take too much imagination to conjure up how that would affect someone's clothing choice for the day. Now, whilst Harry acknowledged this information, he summed it up, scoffed, and declared that it was most definitely T-shirt weather as the sun was out. I once again suggested that Harry take a jumper. 'I'll be right,' came the reply. Back to that later.

Did I mention that we were going to the seaside? I'm not quite sure why I just used the term 'seaside.' Suddenly Enid Blyton comes to mind, and I imagine us having lashings of ginger beer and egg sandwiches on a picnic with Dick and George whilst Timmy the dog barks gleefully at the gulls. Perhaps I was channelling the 'Englishness' of the very good friend whom we were going to visit?

The Mornington Peninsula is quite a familiar destination. To make the most of the journey, I thought we could combine the trip with some business and drop off some information packs to unsuspecting tourism outlets. This was in regard to my latest project, the Australian Adventure Passport. I have been writing kids' books that depict Australian destinations for many years and have just added the Passport to the list. Anyway, the info packs were ready to go and simply needed to be dropped off. I allocated this job to Harry. After much negotiation and because he was freezing, I agreed to buy him a jumper if he delivered some packs. Not quite sure who won with this deal.

Anyway, all went well, and he managed just fine. That was until he met William at one of the tourist outlets. William apparently didn't understand who Harry was and what he was discussing. Harry's attempt to explain to the elderly man was met with confusion and muddled explanations about personal issues, and that he should talk to his bookkeeper, who came on a Friday - or was that Monday? Harry retreated to the safety of the car and firmly declared that he quit. Suddenly, we seemed to be in a Dr. Seuss story.

'I do not like to give these books, I do not like those puzzled looks,
I do not wish to feel annoyed by William, who is paranoid.
I do not like this job at all, now take me to a shopping mall.
I need my jumper and some food, to regain strength and fortitude!'

So, with that, we drove to Sorrento to find something warm for Harry's torso and tum. Now, Sorrento is definitely not the place to find the most cost-effective piece of clothing. However, after attending two university lectures about Economics, Harry was keen to explain to me that purchasing a jumper on sale from $135 to $65 was indeed economically great value. I, of course, pointed out that had he worn a jumper from home, I would have benefited from an even greater economic value!

The Sorrento Hotel provided tasty morsels, excellent company and shelter from the gale-force, Antarctic conditions. We sat in the warmth, smugly protected from the saltwater sprays that were licking the windows and testing the sturdiness of the surrounds.

Alas, lunch eventually ended, and it was time to test our own endurance. For indeed, how can you visit the beach without actually placing a toe on the sand? A half-hearted agreement from me, combined with keener enthusiasm from Harry, saw us meeting the challenge to go for a walk along the shore.

I would estimate that our entire toes-on-sand expedition lasted less than ten minutes. And whilst seagulls and pelicans hovered bravely against the battering wind with fearless determination, and indeed whilst our resolve was strong, we were no match for the Triple Antarctic Blast.

Deciding that sand and sea whipping our legs and scratching our eyes was not at all pleasant, we swiftly escaped to the sanctuary of the car and drove home.

So there you go...

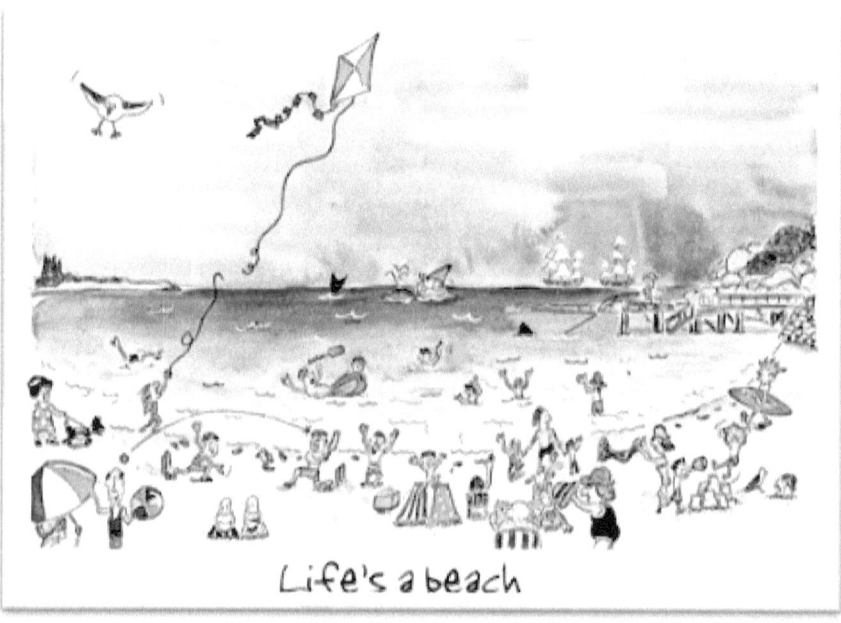

Life's a beach

HYPOTHETICAL CRISIS

At approximately 1:30 pm, on Friday, January 20th, 2017, I was standing on the corner of Flinders and Swanston Street in the city of Melbourne. I had just collected cake decorating supplies from a shop in Port Phillip Arcade to complete my father's 80th birthday cake for celebrations on the coming Sunday. I was outside Young and Jackson's hotel, waiting for the lights to change and cross Flinders when a red vehicle began doing doughies in the intersection. (Anyone unfamiliar, the term doughies refers to a vehicle driving in tight, continuous circles and hence leaving tyre tracks in the shape of a doughnut.)

The driver was the only occupant and was hanging out the window, screaming and clearly upset. My immediate reaction was to move backwards and into the hotel doorway. At that point, I didn't know how serious the situation was; however, I knew I wanted to protect myself and keep an eye on the source of the threat.

At first, there seemed to be confusion from the crowds waiting to cross at the street corners. Some appeared to be entertained by his actions and even admired his driving ability. Many chose to take photos and laugh at what I can only imagine they thought was a daring 'larrikin.' After it was realised that this guy was serious and potentially a dangerous threat, more pedestrians retreated. A few brave souls approached the car and attempted to halt his purpose, unfortunately to no avail. It did cross my mind that a great deal of carnage could have occurred had a firearm been involved. Traffic and trams were halted as police vehicles raced to the scene. The car then sped down Swanston Street towards Bourke Street Mall, where shoppers were gathered.

At that point, I realised that more drama would be likely to unfold, but for now, my day continued.

It was shocking to learn that six people died that day, along with a further twenty-seven who suffered severe injuries from being hit by his car. A drug-induced psychosis was blamed for his reprehensible behaviour. The result is now a city armed with concrete bollards and a wiser notion that we are not immune.

I have met many cancer patients over a multitude of years and have come to understand that everyone finds their own way to deal with their circumstances. I know that my own experiences have altered my coping skills over the years. I have learnt that dealing with facts, rather than hypothetical situations, is sometimes tricky but vital. The unknown is not my department. It creates an often fearful world that can steer me away from the truth and hurl me into unnecessary drama.

So many people on that day in the city of Melbourne, January 2017, will live with the genuine grief, anguish, images and experiences from such a horrific, tragic and pointless violence. They own the tragedy. For myself, whilst I could hypothesise about what may have happened to me if I were standing a block away, buying into that theory is not real. Nothing happened to me. The only emotion I need to deal with is the overwhelming sense of sorrow for those who have been affected.

The observation shouldn't be, '*it could have been me*', but simply be grateful it wasn't.

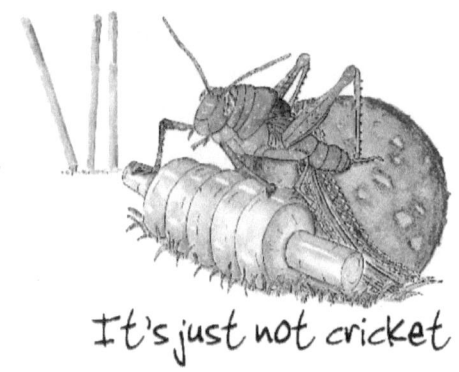

It's just not cricket

Wednesdays with Harry
STREETS WITH NO NAME

Visit Victoria website is full of useful ideas on what to do in Melbourne. There are a series of walks you can download and conduct your own self-guided tours. Today's choice is called Elegant Enclave, a 3km stroll around the classic and rather well-to-do homes of East Melbourne. I did sense that this activity might raise an objection or two from Harry. He explained that, while he couldn't pretend to be joyous, he agreed to partake. Oh, lucky me.

I suggested to Harry to take charge of the map, hoping to encourage his involvement.

'*Mum, I am a bloke; we don't do maps*' he explained.

Yes, of course.

The information included in the guide, to one of us, was fascinating. We wandered along George Street, passing one of Melbourne's oldest homes built in 1856 and discovered the home of Sir Benjamin Benjamin, the Mayor of Melbourne, in the 1880s. Apparently not a typo, his actual name.

At this point, Harry declared that history was boring, and he wished aliens would abduct him to end this torture. Unfortunately for Harry, the streets were void of extraterrestrials, so he had to continue.

So, we crossed Powlett, turned right into Simpson and continued to Hotham, Grey and Gipps. We discovered where Norman Lindsay (Magic Pudding) had courted his first wife, Kate Parkinson and where Picnic at Hanging Rock author Joan Lindsay lived with hubby Daryl. Same spelling, different era and address. We also found the abode of Peter Lalor when he wasn't causing a fracas at the Eureka Stockade.

We followed the map and completed the tour. One of us was pretty entertained by the architecture and history; the other asked,

'*Why do my legs always ache when I am doing something I dislike?*'

Unable to find an answer to such a profound problem, I suggested we retreat to the warmth for lunch.

I was thinking about calling these posts Wednesdays with Harry as a Hostage, but was somewhat heartened when he explained that he actually didn't mind the walk. He just felt like being difficult. Oh, lucky me.

So there you go…

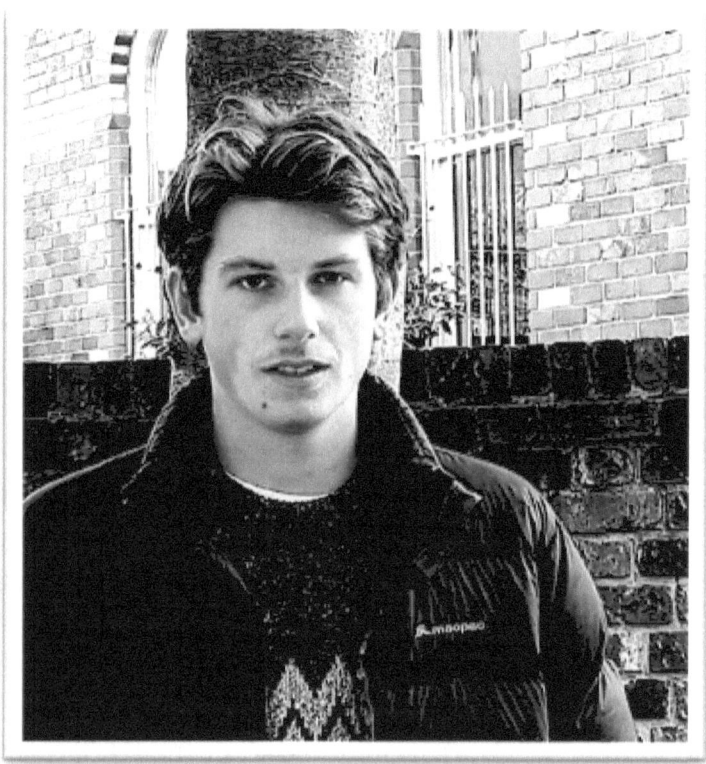

ART THERAPY

Art, what is it? Well, I guess it is many things, but it certainly isn't any images I can put onto paper, or in fact, any other medium. I am the least talented artist on the planet, and if you were wondering who illustrated the artwork in this book, the words are mine, but the images are by Bryce. My laughable attempts at drawing have been validated over many years. Anyone who has played Pictionary with me in the past would have had to rely on mental telepathy rather than the sorry arsed stick figures that I had to offer. So, when I was invited to attend an art therapy session courtesy of a breast cancer organisation, I was a little apprehensive regarding producing a masterpiece. On further inquiry, I was informed that art therapy had little to do with creating an Andy Warhol and everything to do with therapy. I took my chances and went along for the day.

Including myself, there were five attendees at that particular art therapy gathering. The art therapist leading the session presented exactly as one might expect. She was calm, serene, soft and peaceful.

The session began with introductions. I have come to dread when required to discuss and introduce myself to strangers. Usually, the person selected to start this ritual becomes the trailblazer in determining the template for the length of time and amount of detail required. Everyone else then dutifully follows suit. It is a shame they didn't begin with me. On this occasion, the woman who started initiating this ring-a-rosy decided that a ten-minute spiel on her cancer experience was necessary. It was quite a gloomy tale of the stage one breast cancer she had overcome some twenty-five years ago, and clearly, she still held a lot of anger. The following intro spent a little less time explaining her cancer details, but nevertheless gave the impression that she was still mentally affected. I could see where this was all heading, and while I totally respect the outcome of being angry, bitter, and mentally tarnished, I didn't feel like joining in. So, in an attempt to lighten the mood, I only briefly mentioned that I had breast cancer.

Everyone else there had their cancer experiences many years ago. They are survivors. I appeared to be the only one there who didn't quite fit that tag, but really didn't feel the need to explain. It surprised me that these four other women, having left cancer behind years ago, were still sadly affected. But hey, we were all there for therapy.

One of the exercises involved selecting an autumn leaf and gently caressing it whilst drifting into a light meditative state as the instructor calmly directed us to find a tranquil and quiet place in our minds. Returning to the present, we were then handed paper and paint, to use the leaf and incorporate it into some type of art piece. Thankfully, the onus was on abstract. The vision I produced celebrated movement, although that may not have been immediately obvious to the novice. I felt the leaf represented twirling and saw it incorporated as a dancer, perhaps one of ballet. Now, don't be too impressed. The end result was really just a mess of intertwined colours, fighting for the right to spin, whirl and twirl around the autumnal golden amber leaf. I had a squiz at what others were producing and could see that I would not be challenged for the most unusual. The leaf theme was taken literally and inspired pictures of gardens and bouquets—except for one. All I could see was a brown blob.

After enough time and paint had escaped, we were then asked to go around the table again, discussing our art and what we felt when creating. The same woman who took us down the dark cancer path was again the first to discuss. Her image was the brown blob. She explained in quite a lot of detail that the crushed leaf was sprinkled over the dark brown paint, representing the darkness of cancer. I sat and listened with sadness, and I must admit to frustration that someone who had overcome cancer twenty-five years ago was still feeling the need to crush leaves. It is not for me to judge anyone's emotional reactions, so apologies if I sound like I am. I understand entirely the crappiness of cancer, but I also know that holding on to bitterness and anger can be so destructive. It isn't about being constantly 'Pollyanna Positive'; it is about not letting cancer dictate your life. And from what I could ascertain, cancer was still very much up front and centre. It was winning. If I have the privilege of still being here in twenty-five years, I can guarantee I will be bursting with gratitude and appreciation and definitely not crushing leaves with brown paint.

The other observation I have concerning the anger directed at cancer is that cancer cells are my cells. We often talk about cancer as if it is some type of alien creature that dared to infiltrate our bodies in the dark of night. It is my cells that have been out to party, and whilst they may appear to have malicious intent, they are made from me. If they are rebellious, then that I am. Hating these cells is hating me. I may feel incredibly frustrated about what has happened to my health, but being angry at what my own body has created is not helpful.

Obviously, anger is such a subjective topic regarding cancer. I have met many people with cancer who are very angry about their situation, as are their loved ones. I would expect if someone I loved was affected by such a crappy disease, I too would hold some resentment.

I guess our own individual perspective on life determines our outlook towards dealing with something like cancer. To me, the knowledge that there are so many people genuinely suffering and fighting to actually survive, far outweighs anything I have yet to go through. And, if ever I am grappling with feeling a little overwhelmed, I think of Slater Walker, who passed away in August 2021. He was six years old. Slater was diagnosed with brain cancer when he was only seventeen months old. It is heartbreaking that any child suffers from cancer. In Slater's case, well, the fact that his entire life was hideously riddled with the full crappiness of cancer is simply shattering. Brain cancer kills more children here in Australia than any other disease. I cannot imagine how difficult it would be for the child, parents and family involved. If you ever want to talk about inspiration and courage, then look no further than Slater Walker.

Well, the art therapy session ended, and we all went on our way, proudly carrying our creations.

Was it useful? The fact that I am writing about it years later suggests there was plenty to take away. Whilst I endeavour to reduce cancer's clout by attempting to leave it in the corner, I think it is terrific that those going through or have gone through experiences with cancer have the opportunities to congregate, compare, discuss and express their emotions.

I am not cancer. I am simply a really dreadful artist who aspires to win at Pictionary.

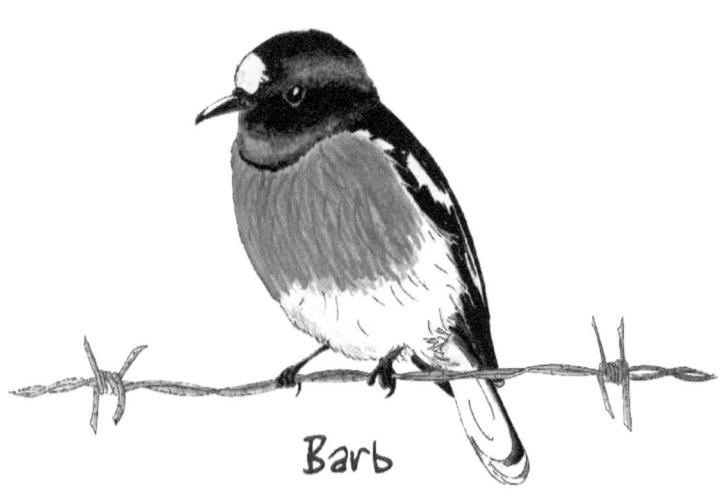

Wednesdays with Harry
HOLD THE PHONE

Some days, no matter how well-intentioned you are to achieve greatness, you just get bogged down in other stuff. Today was one of those days, and so my grandiose plans have been put on hold, of course, much to Harry's extreme disappointment. The 'stuff' I refer to has left my brain shattered, my patience tested, my will to live slim and with a sizable headache.

The day began with the appropriate degree of enthusiastic zest as I phoned the Australian Tax Office at precisely 9:00 am. On hold for an hour and forty minutes left me questioning the need to have a chat, so I changed tactics and called the superannuation company in relation to my query. After thirty minutes of repeatedly pressing #2 for a consultant, I was finally connected to an actual person.

Sharon had a pleasant enough personality, though my question caused her to put me on hold for an additional twenty minutes while she researched the answer. Then it was established that she needed to transfer me to Marnie, who would undoubtedly be a helpful ally. Marnie was also friendly enough; however, after another fifteen minutes, she decided to return me to Sharon to complete the request. Eventually, both Sharon and Marnie concluded that my query was a little too difficult, but they enthusiastically suggested I phone the ATO to follow up. Of course!

Meanwhile, Harry pushed me to follow up with the postal service regarding his Nikes I had purchased online for his birthday. His birthday was at the beginning of April, so they were running a tad late. I discovered that it had arrived in Australia in mid-April and was passed on to the local postal service to continue its journey. The tracking number stated it was *'On its way'*. I now realise that the post is currently delayed due to Covid and everyone's need to shop online; nevertheless, I thought they might be able to identify where it was and how long it would take to arrive. Failing to discover a phone number, I had no option but to use their online chat thingy.

It began by connecting me to a robot dude who, sorry to say, was no help with an individual query. I was then given the option to wait for the 'Live chat' consultant. It informed me that I was #28 in the queue. Yay.

Finally, David textually introduced himself and explained that the post was delayed, but they were doing their best. Yes, I understood that and complimented their hard work, but I still questioned why the tracking number hadn't updated the information since April 14. He explained again that they were very busy and not everything was scanned, but it would be *'On its way'*. Yes, I understood that, but surely the idea of a tracking number means that you can actually track it and could tell me its whereabouts. David then explained that they were very busy and overloaded with mail, but they were doing their best, and he was certain my parcel would be in transit. I asked about the transport, and he told me that it would be on a truck. Yes, David, but where exactly was this truck? David then explained that they were very busy and doing their best to cope with the increase in mail. I began to wonder if David was, in fact, a Live Chat person and not an incognito robot, but gave him the benefit of the doubt. Finally, I was defeated, and so, after an hour and a half, I had had enough of this runaround and informed Harry that the postal service was working very hard, and hopefully, his Nikes were *'On their way!'*

To add to my day, at precisely 2:43 p.m., the internet dropped out. Yes, did the usual reboot and verbally abused the whole communication system before searching for any outages in our area. Nope, not the issue. And so, after pressing every relevant button, I took a deep breath and summoned up the strength to call the telecommunication company. After being on hold for what felt like an eternity, I finally gave up and found the microscopic hole in the modem, then shoved a paperclip in. The modem took about twenty minutes to decide if I had buggered it completely or was happy to reconnect. Fortunately, it was the latter, and we are now happily back in the world of the web with minimum inconvenience.

Now I realise my day is not that unusual, and we are all subjected to such days. Good on you for handling it better than I.

Fortunately, phones have speakers, and so whilst on hold, I did manage to do the washing, sweep the floor, wash the dishes, wash my hair, watch Dancing with Wolves, bake sausage rolls, eat the sausage rolls, grow a plum tree and performed surgery on my toe - so not a complete waste of a day!

So there you go...

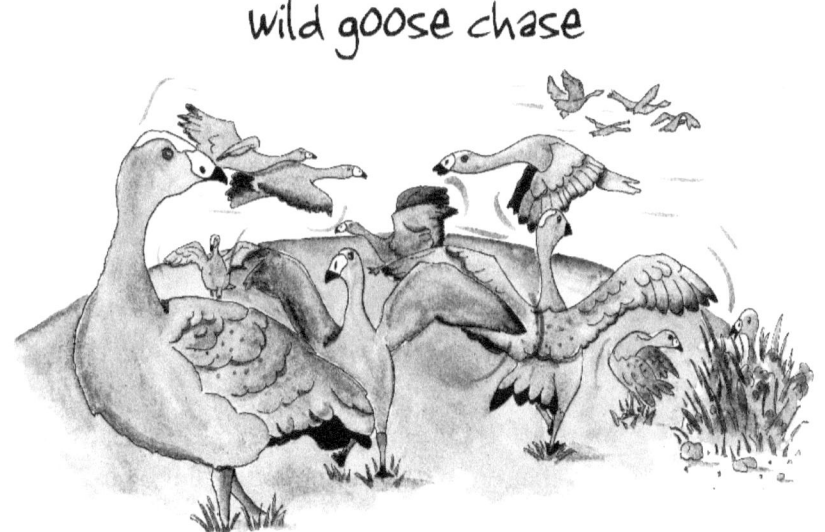

wild goose chase

APPRAISING THE FUNDRAISING

It was October 2015, still in chemo treatment. I was about to enter a supermarket when I noticed a breast cancer fundraising table set up, fully decked out with the appropriate pink signature pamphlets and paraphernalia. The person manning the stall managed to catch my eye and stopped me for a chat. He began to inform me about the high rates of breast cancer and the much-needed fundraising to help eradicate it in the future. This wasn't the first time I had been stopped in such a situation, and I knew that interrupting his spiel would be pointless. The offer on the table was to commit to a monthly donation. Finally, I explained that, while I understand and thoroughly applaud his fundraising efforts, I wasn't currently in a financial position to commit to a monthly deduction. He pressed me a little further and explained that it would be likely that someone I loved would one day be affected by breast cancer, and how I could help by donating today.

At that point, it occurred to me that my quest to *chase normal* was working. It didn't seem noticeable how tired I felt nor the lopsidedness of my chest or, in fact, that my hair was replaced with a synthetic wig. So I did find myself in a quandary. Do I remain incognito, or do I disclose my own health issues and enter the conversation from the point of view of a person with cancer?

I could see that he wasn't going to let go too quickly and so simply explained that I was currently going through chemo for breast cancer, and I greatly appreciate all that fundraising can do. He then told me that he was so sorry that I was going through that, but I must have been coping with the chemo just fine as I looked so well. He added that I should be even keener to help since I was in that situation. I thanked him again and then had the urge to explain a little further.

Perhaps not only to validate my reasons for not donating, but also to create awareness for others.

It makes total sense that those affected by cancer would want to donate the most towards the cause, but the reality is that the financial situation of such cases is often already stretched. I rationalised to him that whilst the physical and mental issues are generally at the top of the stress list involving cancer, financial hardships are possibly something that could also be impacting a person or family going through cancer. Having treatment often meant giving up working, so a drop in finances was often another added anxiety. Those diagnosed with more advanced cancers faced not only an uncertain future with treatments and, in fact, life itself, but also with finances. Families supporting are also stretched.

I didn't want to bang on about it, so I apologised for not being able to donate right then and again thanked him for his time and commitment. He said he understood and wished me the best.

We are so lucky to have most treatments supported by government assistance in this country. Still, unfortunately, the need to also have an income, regardless of diagnosis, often means finances become strained. It is a great pity that private fundraising is necessary for medical advances. One day, perhaps, we will have governments unite across the globe with the sole purpose of totally committing financially to researching cures for cancers and other such diseases.

It also raises the topic of which types of cancer receive more fundraising or funding. Personally, I think that cancer is cancer. I don't look at the colour of the ribbon it represents. To me, there is really only curable or incurable cancer. I know that most funding and research goes into early detected cancers because it is there that we can win. The future for many can look brighter, which is a great thing. For those of us with metastatic cancers, we can only hang on and hope that funds can also be applied and advances also made. Hope is really all we often have.

On that day in October 2015, I was unable to afford a donation, and whilst over the years it hasn't added up to much, I have donated where I can. I know family and friends have also done the same. It does seem that so many of the fundraisers and campaigns are initiated by family and friends who have known or know someone with cancer. It becomes personal and is done with passion.

If this is you, please know that you are an angel of outstanding quality, and your efforts are wholeheartedly treasured.

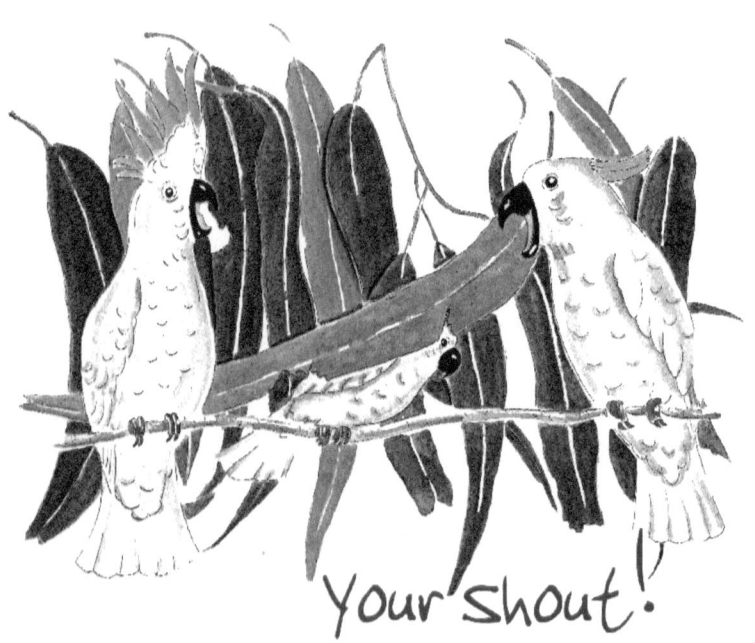

Wednesdays with Harry
PAINT BY NUMBERS

Well, exams are over and survived - not sure yet if thrived, however, what will be will be. Regular discussions have occurred around the idea of Harry gaining employment for the summer. Now when I say 'discussions,' that actually equates to me rabbiting on and Harry vaguely acknowledging he is listening. He does work one day a week at a tennis club, which is fabulous, but that leaves six days left in the week to account for until university starts again.

Perhaps it is the influence of watching renovation programs or the fact that Dulux was offering a can of jellybeans with paint purchases, but Harry's counter to this employment suggestion was offering to paint the house. Yes, it is sadly overdue, and the colours selected ten years ago are perhaps a little tired, and so I agreed.

Now let's face it, nobody enjoys painting, well certainly not me, even though it appears contrary to that fact as I have had the task in the past to cover every wall, ceiling, floor, window frame, chair and cupboard. There was no escape. I had mastered the brush and roller, succumbed to the latest trends, created suede effect feature walls, conquered the art of cutting in, designed painted patterns on the floor and impulsively updated and altered colours as my mood dictated.

Well, that was a decade ago. Lymphedema in my right arm and neuropathy in my hands and feet has left me somewhat incapacitated to wield a brush without considerable consequences. So, the house and I have taken a very long breath and learnt to relax and accept the colours that be. Any spontaneous urges to alter the tints, hues and style have been quashed, and the rollers have retired to a dark corner of the shed where they have sadly surrendered to crustiness and rust.

Therefore, Harry's suggestion to paint the house was readily accepted.

Day one of painting in tradies' terms would quite likely mean prising open the lid of the sparkling new paint tin early morning. I was up and dressed in appropriate paint coaching attire and sat with anticipation beside paint, new rollers and brushes as I waited for my very own 'tradie' to arise from his slumber. Eventually, he surfaced and explained that he still needed to go for a run, shower, eat breakfast and read the paper before work could possibly begin. I said to Harry that is not how tradies work. He explained to me that this is precisely why he is going to university and chooses not to be one. At exactly 1 pm, Harry attempted to release the lid on the paint tin…with a stick. This task appeared to be the first stumbling block, and at that point, I realised I needed to locate old paint-worthy clothes, put aside thoughts of inflammation and help get some paint on the walls.

I would like to say that we worked well together; however, that would be quite an exaggeration. The issue seemed to be that I believed I had some experience and knowledge and began to advise Harry on how to hold a brush, how much paint to put on the roller, how to cut in, which ladder to use, why he needed to lay down a drop sheet, why he shouldn't stand on the couch with paint on his feet, how long to leave the paint tape in place and why he should clean up paint that had dripped on the floor due to misplaced drop sheet as soon as possible - and Harry seemed to believe that none of this information was necessary.

The differences of opinion continued until I found myself shuffling along on my rear end, painting architraves, and discovered that I couldn't seem to get off the floor. With a cramp in one leg and spasms in my side, I suggested that I might need some help getting up. Finally, Harry agreed and rallied to winch me off the floor.

Fortunately, we also agreed on the type of music. Music is quite often a welcome mediator.

You may be surprised to know that we have now managed to spread the paint in the general vicinity of the walls in a few rooms and hallway. Almost halfway, and then there is the outside. I'm not sure my aching body will cope with much more, and as for Harry's input, I'm actually very proud of his efforts and persistence in doing a good job.

He hasn't managed to start before midday yet, but there you go…

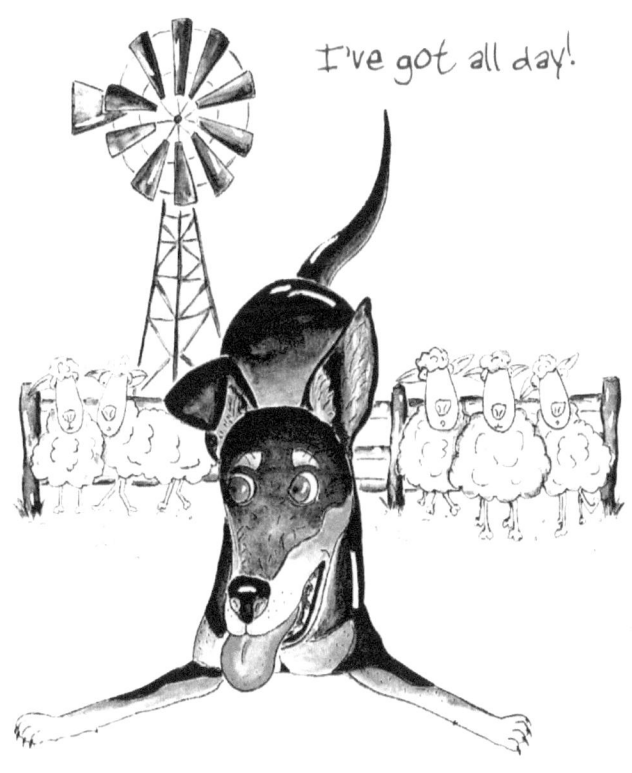

TRIAL AND ERROR

February 10th, 2020

Regular scans are always followed up with an appointment with my oncologist to discuss the results. Waiting is never easy, and trepidation is always present, but with every 'status quo' result comes the hope that everything will continue as it is. On this particular day, it didn't.

I was told that cancer had progressed. Several doctors had conferred and mutually agreed that the nodules on my lungs had grown. The progression of cancer meant that my current tolerated targeted treatment would need to be changed. It was also noted that the nodules were now large enough to biopsy. Therefore, I was presented with two options. One was to participate in a clinical trial. Clinical trials undergo various stages before being released for public use, and this trial was in phase three. If it was deemed successful, phase four would finalise it before being released as an approved drug. Like most chemotherapies, the side effects were potentially extreme, as was the intense scrutiny process. It was also a randomised controlled study comparing the results with a drug that was the current option. This means I may have been administered the trial drug or the currently used alternative drug. The alternative to participating in the clinical trial was to use the drug being compared. Either way, it was full-on soul-destroying chemo again with all the bells and whistles.

I have endured this type of chemotherapy twice before, but always with an end date in mind. Whilst I am in treatment every three weeks and have been told that it will be for the rest of my life, it is currently a targeted treatment, and I tolerate it well. This time, I would need to remain on chemo until cancer progresses again and then another until there are no more treatment options available or, indeed, my body can't cope. My interpretation - it was the beginning of the end.

The conversation with the oncologist was reasonably practical and matter-of-fact, as there has always been the underlying assumption that this day would come. Not assumed by me, however. Being confronted with cancer is not a place I choose to visit. The fear I felt that cancer was now winning was just like the first time all over again. I would have thought, after all these years, that I would be somehow immune to its power. The numbness kicked in, and I didn't respond at all emotionally. I sat and tried to understand the clinical trial process and agreed that it was probably the best course of action. I was then booked for a further appointment with the trial personnel in a few days.

I have often prattled on about accepting things you cannot change, and the quicker you get there, the more balanced you can remain. Every time I am challenged with the prognosis that my life is coming closer to the end, it throws me off balance, and I question everything. I try to hang onto the knowledge that thoughts cannot hurt me, *'the past doesn't exist, it's just memories in the present, the future doesn't exist, it's just thoughts in the present'* so stay present. However, the reality was that I left that appointment with the twenty-four pages of clinical trial information and a feeling of despair. An emotional tantrum was brewing, and I wanted to scream into some dark abyss that I was not going to die.

I felt like I was waiting at a bus stop, except I was unsure which bus I needed to catch. I needed to decide quickly as I had checked the schedule, and the first bus was due to arrive shortly. This bus would be full of cancer patients along with masked, gowned and gloved medical staff who will beckon me on board and offer a seat up front. But this seat comes with a catch. Whilst you would be allowed to know exactly where you are heading, the view was clouded by the reality and loneliness of mortality. Chemotherapy was the treatment offered. It would be unfriendly, debilitating, relentless, and uncompromising, with no end in sight. It was predicted that I would continue on this journey for a while, but there was no doubt about its final destination. This bus would not return to the station. It would just keep driving until the fuel was exhausted and come to a spluttering, defeated end.

I sat in my car and tried to get my brain to function. A good friend was working close by, and so I called, and we met to discuss. I needed more rational minds than my own to offer some sensible advice.

There was a mutual emotional reaction after she had read the information. That conversation also allowed me to hear my inner voice. That intuitive voice that is always there, sometimes quietly nagging but always offering to lead the way. It told me that I needed to pull back from the trial, and in fact, all suggested treatment until I had a biopsy. Delaying treatment to wait for a biopsy was purely based on trusting my instincts. The best way to know if you can trust something is simply to trust it.

So I found myself dangling precariously on a tightrope between the hopeful naivety of denial and the harsh medical understanding of reality. It was all I could do to cling to my instinctive belief in having trust. Perhaps that meant that I had to let the first bus pass and wait for another.

The second bus wasn't running on time; in fact, it was notorious for its tardiness and erratic route choices. On board, I was greeted by the idea that I could fully contribute to my own destiny by taking charge of my own path. Long, winding roads lay ahead, allowing for the discovery of inner strength, knowledge, freedom, and joy. This bus may, in fact, run alongside the first bus, but it ultimately steers its own course. The destination of this bus is unknown.

The truth be known, I am not brave. I just wanted to pull a blanket over my head and believe that this was truly a bad dream, and I would wake up and look forward to a long and healthy future. Instead, I took quiet steps towards what my instincts told me, immersed myself in knowledge, reignited the will to live and tried to remain rational.

I involved more family and friends and ultimately decided to ask for a biopsy. I then watched reruns of *Taskmaster (UK)* because distraction and humour is always a good idea.

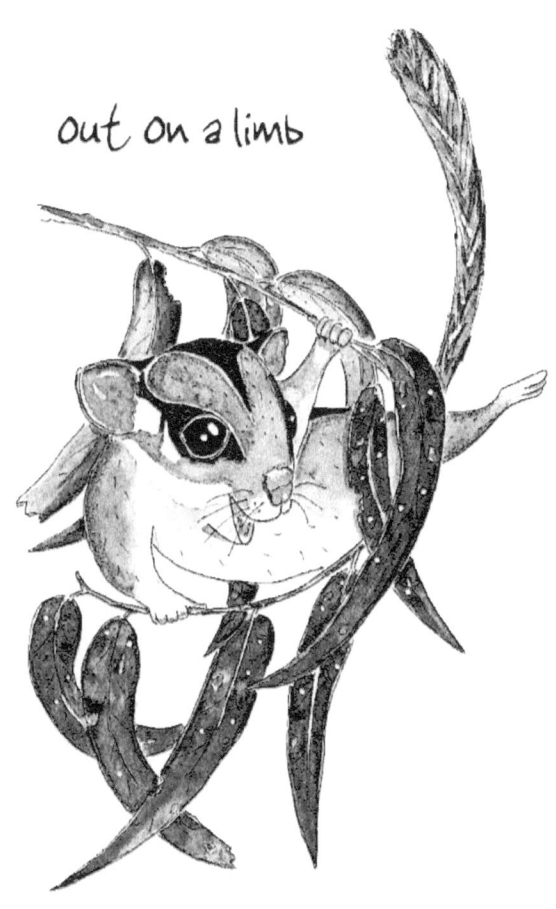

Wednesdays with Harry
GRUMPY OLD WOMAN

University exams are underway, which means Harry is locked in his room, teetering on the brink of extinction as I slide food under the door and just assume the mumbled grunt of thanks is actually him in there toiling away. Of course, conducting an exam at home over forty-eight hours with open books is a far cry from white knuckles penning answers feverishly in an exam room onsite.

Earlier in the week, we did manage to go on an outing together, albeit to the supermarket. Waiting for our freedom to travel more than 5 km in Covid is taking its toll, and now that we are allowed more than one shopper per household, Harry jumped at the opportunity to come with me and do the weekly shop. It was our first outing together in months; I could sense the delight and excitement.

It has come to my attention that shopping with Harry inevitably increases the total expense. The trolley begins to fill with men's toiletries, protein balls and far too many avocados, and why would I object to four-dollar packets of pea-flavoured corn chips? The extra help does come in handy, however, not just in unloading and reloading at the checkout, but also as a decoy from the unavoidable chit-chat that is about to probe into my personal life from the lovely, young and far too happy checkout person.

Of course, I realise I should be beholden and grateful that millennials feel the need to chat with me at all, but I simply don't wish to explain how busy I have been today, what I plan to do after shopping, and what I do for a living. Therefore, I begin to make futile conversation with Harry, and I sense that he is onto my strategy. This was immediately confirmed by him saying, '*Mum, I am onto your strategy*'.

I can see the power quickly going to his head, and his challenging grin threatens to ignore me completely. Through somewhat ventriloquistic skills, I explain that I will hold the pea chips hostage unless he obliges. Mum wins.

Now, this leads me to the abhorrent realisation that I have indeed reached the age and disposition of a grumpy old woman - and yes, I am internally groaning at the thought.

The evidence: I would rather cosy up beside reruns of *The Great British Bake Off* than go out for dinner; I prefer comfort over fashion; I have serious issues with anyone fitting the loo roll on the wrong way – yes, there is a right way; I am quite intolerant of idiots; I have a tough time when the youth, or in fact anyone, use the word '*like*' fourteen times in one sentence; I seem to say '*when I was your age*' regularly; it irritates me that my hair is thinning, that everything sags and I cannot read the fine print, in fact, any print without glasses or contacts; I find myself contemplating the need to buy anti-wrinkle products and go to sleep with bits of silicone strips adhered to my face; it annoys me that young people look young, and I genuinely believe the most valuable possession I own is a good pair of tweezers. In fact, generally, I find myself annoyed about being annoyed!

Ahh, the joys of aging gracefully.

So there you go…

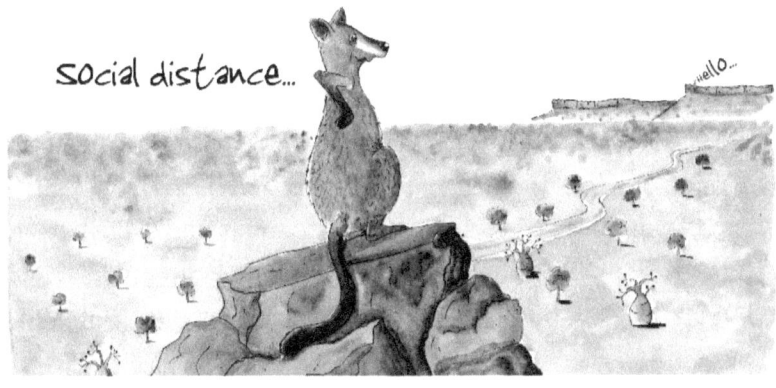

LIVE TO FLIGHT ANOTHER DAY

March 5th, 2020

The lung biopsy was not particularly enjoyable, but in my mind, undoubtedly necessary. The preparation before this procedure was much like many others. Assigned a bed and cubicle, changed into a well-worn hospital gown, possessions housed in a blue plastic basket, portacath accessed, vitals taken, forms completed, doctors chatted, potential dangers discussed. The biopsy meant that a scan would be monitoring the position of the nodules, so definitely no moving whilst a medical instrument would be inserted through my back and into my lungs. This would be repeated a few times until all samples were taken, or indeed my lung collapsed or bled. Yay.

I had no second thoughts and thoroughly trusted the surgeon's expertise. This time, my sister was with me and had the task of keeping me company and enduring the usual wait time. All good. Lungs behaved well and continued to function as they should.

The results came in about a week later. I had no real expectations that it wouldn't be cancer; but as it had been nine years since first diagnosed, I wanted to confirm that the treatment in place suited this particular type of cancer.

Personalised treatment is vitally needed in this country. From my perspective, the *'one size fits all'* approach is fraught with issues. Precision Medicine is one of the most significant overall advances in how cancer is treated. Understanding the makeup of your particular cancer cells and receiving the most appropriate treatment is a game-changer. Incorrect treatment means that precious time is wasted, with unnecessary side effects occurring, and even lives are lost. Check out **Love Your Sister**'s website and appreciate the significant fundraising and awareness they are undertaking to encourage Precision Medicine as the standard care for all Australians.

It is difficult to express the relief I felt when I was told that those nodules were not cancer but inflammation. I was also informed that it was plausible that the nodules tested were not the cancerous ones, and so progression was still a possibility. Phooey!

As it turned out, however, I am quite the exception. I am not sure how unique I am, but I know that my instincts to have a biopsy were validated. It has also made me sit up and question more, educate myself more and demand more answers before I agree to more harmful treatment. It highlighted not only the critical role my instincts play but also my responsibility and accountability for my own health.

Whilst it hasn't changed my advanced metastatic prognosis, and my regular three weekly targeted treatment will continue, it has meant I can breathe again - relief is an obvious reaction, along with the understanding that we were all given gut instincts for a reason.

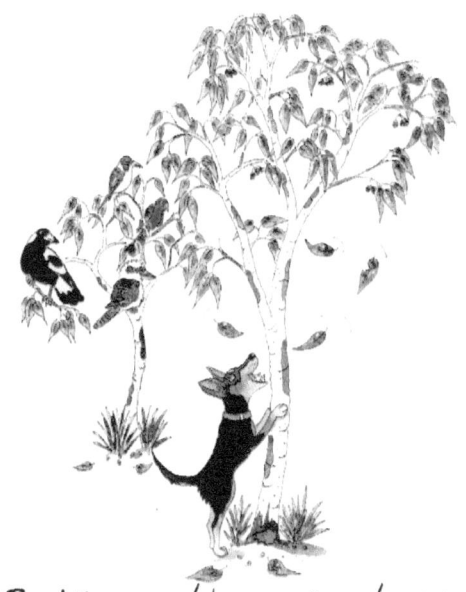

Barking up the wrong tree

Wednesdays with Harry
HAPPY 21ST

April 8th, 2020

Well, it took Harry to turn twenty-one and a little forced isolation for my board game fervour to be allowed to surface from the depths of priority. And in fact, it is two days later, and the game of choice is still set up on the dining room table. I fear, however, that it says more about lethargy to pack it up rather than Harry's newfound excitement and motivation to continue to play.

Currently, the screeching noise from the new F1 PlayStation game strongly indicates revving the turbocharged vehicle, steering it into a slipstream after dragging out from pole position, all from the comfort of the couch cockpit, is seemingly overtaking the desire to pursue trivia in a board game.

So, my one and only child reached the age of twenty-one. He does declare confusion as to why it is such a milestone, especially as he became an adult at eighteen. I'm not sure which particular definition of an adult should be used at eighteen, and in fact, I know fifty-year-olds who are still searching for that description, but I concede that I understand what he means. I advise him to put it down to tradition and just go with it. Of course, the fact that we are stuck at home in isolation doesn't help sell the party theory that tradition requires a big shindig. I acknowledge that the celebrations I had hoped for were likely a reflection of my own need to mark the milestones. No matter how positive I feel regarding my health, there is always a tiny nagging doubt that I will miss out on all of the big stuff.

Harry didn't seem to mind that the celebrations were relatively mild, but I asked for contributions towards a video I was compiling for him to try and compensate. Thanks to more than sixty messages, from primary school teachers, footy and tennis coaches, to friends, family, and others, that kept him guessing, I was able to record a memorable keepsake that he really appreciated.

Now, just when you thought his day couldn't get any more wrapped up in motherly love, I presented him with a one hundred-and eighty-seven-page bound edition of Wednesdays with Harry - the story so far. He looked a little overwhelmed at the prospect, so I thought it prudent to gently guide and motivate him to understand the correct response upon receiving such a book. Much to Harry's delight, ahem, for the next little while, we sat and relived some memories and revisited outings.

By now, you may be feeling sorry for Harry, as he was being forced into sentimental torture on his special day. Pleased to say that he acted interested and laughed and guffawed in all the correct places. So, there you go, a little prompting and nagging can open the door to forty-four thousand words of joy!

Enough sentimental gifts, it was time to pull out the big guns and give him presents he actually wanted.

The afternoon was spent playing Trivial Pursuit – yes, his choice! I tried to insist on partaking in beer pong, but Harry informed me quite emphatically that it would be just too weird to play drinking games with his mum. To be honest, I am well out of practice, and so we settled for a bottle of champagne whilst trying to recall if Ronald Reagan and Gorbachev met at a summit conference in Iceland? Interestingly enough, the more I drank, the less I knew, which seemed in complete contrast to Harry. His intelligence oddly improved with consumption.

Happy Birthday was sung, candles were blown out, the cake was cut, and the remains were still being eaten. Streamers and balloons are now sagging and deflated, yet defiantly hanging on to extend their stay and remind us of the party that was.

Thanks to all those who helped make Harry's day special.

Wednesdays with Harry

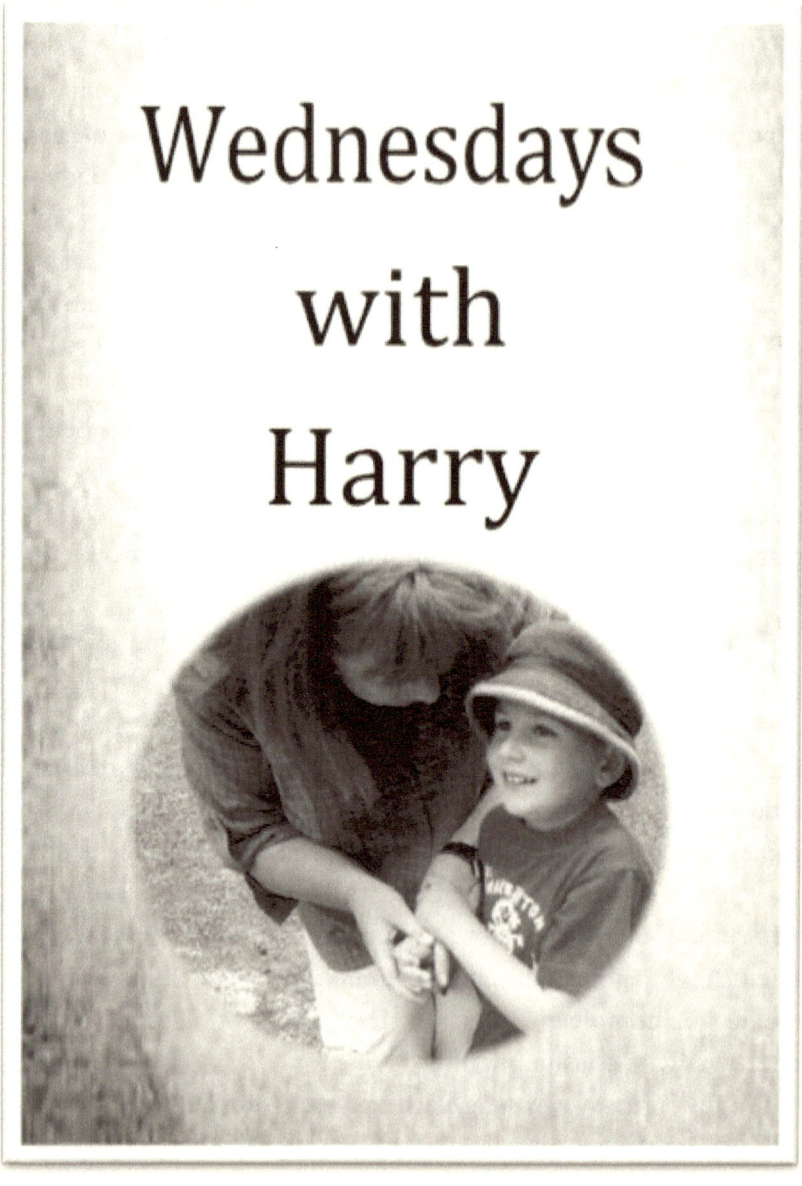

TIRED

Today is one of those days - I'm tired. It starts off feeling tired and ends much the same. Not the sort of tiredness that comes from lack of sleep or being overworked, but the type of tired that seeps out of every pore, bone and fibre. It's as if tired invited its brothers, sisters and cousins, and they have all come to sit on my shoulders. They unite in their quest to exhaust and drain the last shred of energy until fatigue and lethargy dominate. The weight is pressing. My eyes struggle to remain open, and my brain is left to declare insufficient deposits to function. The luxury of staying in bed and succumbing is tempting.

The attributes of this variety of tiredness extend beyond simply weariness. It is typically accompanied by heightened pain and emotional distress. The peripheral neuropathy that has found a home in my hands and feet tends to burn more and guarantees the complete absence of fine motor skills.

I stand and stare at an unopened tube of mayonnaise and begin to wonder if Occupational Therapists make house calls. Solving the issue of opening mayonnaise became too much of a challenge, and I began to feel frustrated. Should I really waste feeling sorry for myself over a tube of mayonnaise? Surely, I should save that for something more substantial? So, I toss the mayonnaise aside and smash open an avocado instead. The solutions are not what they used to be. Years ago, I would have tackled that tube with strength, fortitude and a non-quitter attitude.

Who am I kidding? Days like these are an emotional ticking time bomb, and I'm looking for anything to light the fuse. The annoying twitch from nerve damage in my left eyebrow starts pulsating, and I wonder if that is worthy of emotional distress. The fact that I am logically ascertaining whether that is indeed the case suggests that I am simply seeking emotional validation. It's not necessary.

Cancer provides that justification anytime I need it. It is the golden ticket to a sentimental, temperamental, demonstrative self-pity and melancholy party, and no one would think any less. Do I use that ticket? Very rarely.

On so many levels, cancer can be tiring. But here is the thing - I am very aware that I really only have one trick up my sleeve, which is to deny cancer that right. That right to dominate and control.

I do have days when I feel anxious and downhearted, and where sorrow and despondency are present, and that's okay.

Today is one of those days - I'm tired.

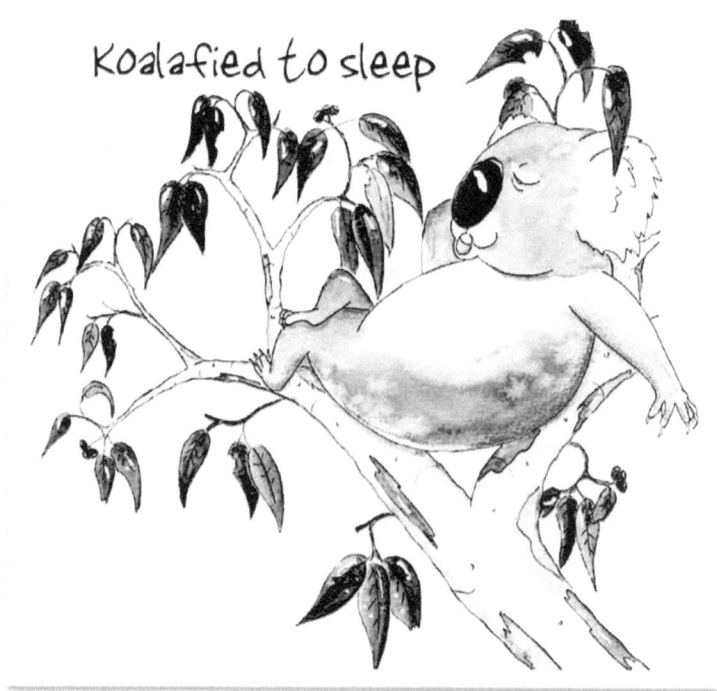

Wednesdays with Harry
CINEMATIC JOY

This week I managed to drag Harry away from various activities and convinced him to join me in watching a film - AT AN ACTUAL CINEMA.

It seems an eternity ago that viewing a film at the cinema was a standard form of entertainment. If you wished to watch a new release before six months after it became available on Video or DVD, then you had no choice but to frequent the cinema. Of course, if you knew someone visiting Bali, you may well have jumped the queue with a perfectly dodgy copy of the latest blockbuster, complete with audience participation. You could enjoy the film wearing your Rolex watch, sporting some Air Jordans and holding a Gucci handbag.

Now, going to the cinema is more than just arousing the passion of film; it is the entire excursion that makes it worthwhile. Whilst I am sure many moviegoers still appreciate the effort of watching a movie on the big screen, it seems to have taken a back seat to flicking on the TV. Our choice of media shifts with technology. Tossed aside were the outdated videos for the more durable DVDs. However, my DVD library, which once stood proudly in uniform, catalogued rows, is now lying quite obsolete on a dusty shelf. Foxtel, Netflix and Stan have landed and have satisfied the instant gratification we seem to have for fulfilling our needs RIGHT NOW.

Of course, there are flaws in this modern movie-watching experience. Our insatiable appetites are overwhelmed by the number of really crappy movies that are instantly available, and we can spend precious movie-watching time deciding which one to watch. However, the most obvious failing is that it leaves us still in our lounge rooms, removed from social interactions and the sheer joy of an outing.

There is something quite fulfilling about watching a film in a cinema. You are transported entirely, surrounded by sight and sound that hold your full attention. For the next two hours, there will be no distractions, no noise and thoughts other than what is before you, and I can't tell you how much I needed that right now. You are contained in a theatre, sink into your seat and surrender to the big screen. Then there is always that moment of confusion when exiting a cinema. You emerge from the dark and are pretty shocked to find that it is now raining and that you are not actually in Africa, having your hair washed by Robert Redford, but instead, you are adjusting to your new surroundings and wondering where you left the car.

Now, back to our outing, and I insisted we go to the glorious Art Deco Rivoli Cinema. Harry did not understand my choice of cinema and declared that the building, being an art deco structure, could not possibly alter the movie experience. He is mistaken. The Rivoli is a magnificent building. On entering, you are immediately transported back to the glory days of cinema, complete with appropriately themed 40's music playing in the foyer and throughout the loos. Ahh, bliss. Well, it would be bliss if we weren't running really late and then had to contend with a very long queue of school kids lining up for popcorn and tickets to the latest kids' flick. It is not our thing to be on time for anything, but when it's an occasion where it will start without us, my penetrating glare at the limited number of staff selling tickets immediately goes into action. Please, POLLEEESSE, will the fussy kid and indeed his pampering mother, please decide between M&Ms or Maltesers – NOW! We are in a hurry and don't have time for you to deliberate, discuss, and ponder the pros and cons of chocolate choices.

Fortunately, the preshow advertising was the only bit we missed. We found our seats, and it became immediately apparent that we were two of five people attending this film. I am not quite sure why you need a nominated seat number these days; however, I would suggest that seating the entire audience side by side is really not necessary. Not one to particularly pay attention to such rules, we found alternative seats where we didn't need to fight for the armrest or cup holder. Harry felt that the fact that there were only five of us was a reflection of the film's watchability. Nonsense. It was purely because everyone else had already seen it.

The Green Book. One of the best films I have seen in quite a while. An emotional trapeze. The fine line between digesting the deplorable, instinctive humour, raw sensibilities and simple human kindness was just perfect. A brilliant film based on a true story, enhanced by some outstanding acting. And hey, even Harry agreed.

My cinema experience has been reignited, and just like the rebirth of the vinyl record, I can hang on to the hope that everything old is new again. Long live the cinema!

So there you go…

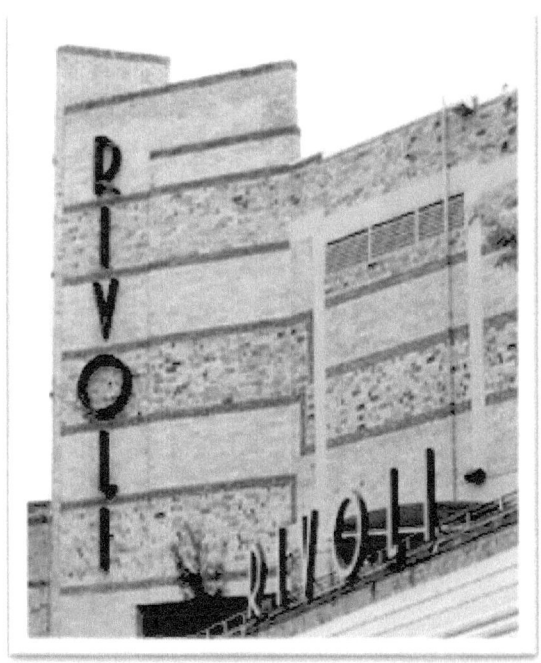

ONCOLOGY ANGELS

Every year since 1965, on May 12th, International Nurses Day has been celebrated. I doubt the celebrations stretch to a day off and kicking up heels, as there is simply too much work to be done. The date is significant as it is the anniversary of Florence Nightingale's birth. Every year, a theme for this recognition is presented, and this year is *A Vision for the Future*. With Covid-19 still raging, it must be difficult to find clarity in such a vision.

I am writing this from the oncology ward where I frequent every three weeks. In the days before Covid-19, it would have been likely that one or two family members would have popped in for a visit. They adapted to the routine, put the dates in their diaries, and would come to create opportunities to keep up with all the family gossip. I think it also helped them to feel connected. My quest for independence over the years has often meant that my family has felt helpless and only as involved or helpful as I allow. I know it isn't easy for them, but I do know that retaining independence gives me strength.

On some occasions, Harry would also come with me. The interest for Harry would be minimal at best, and I give him credit for at least attempting to humour me. I may jest and emphasise his indifference and his seeming lack of interest, his monotone mutterings and general apathy. By the way, he assures me that he saves most of that just for me! Of course, much of that is somewhat broad generational commentary. I do, in fact, love his self-motivation, determination, sporting prowess, commitment to a cause, quirky outlook, and choice of socks. His dry sense of humour is very much like mine, and we laugh often. While many of his characteristics do align with the 'typical' teenager or young adult stereotype, he also offers a unique and fundamental perspective on life. His unembellished yet naturally droll perspective is often precisely what I need, and in many ways, he is my saviour. I am truly blessed.

We are currently going through quite an unusual and somewhat challenging time with the Covid pandemic, and many feel overwhelmed by the situation. I am doing okay, pandemically speaking, but then again, I have had years of experience in health matters. We do need to adapt to change, and it is entirely your choice which attitude you select. Of course, there is no particular joy in having metastatic cancer, but it has given me a perspective on life that somehow allows me to sift through the unnecessary stuff. Anyway, I mention this today because I feel the need to wholeheartedly thank the staff and particularly Deb, Nicki, Lisa, and Sam, who have been my nurses here for too many years to count. They are the most amazing women who tackle all their tasks with such care and patience. Undoubtedly, they are challenged with the emotions that naturally spill into an oncology ward, but they handle it all with thoughtfulness and a sensitivity that is so important. International Nurses Day is next week, and among all frontline workers, I believe nurses deserve recognition and gratitude.

I know that I could never have been a nurse; not only would I be grimacing and most likely chundering at the sight or smell of bodily emissions, but I would simply not have the tolerance or empathy that is clearly required. They are not just doing a job; they are invested in every patient that crosses their path. Patients become personalities they come to know, and for whatever amount of time they are in their care, they laugh, celebrate, cry and feel with us and for us.

We currently use the term *'we are all in this together,'* but nowhere else I know truly emulates that saying, as in the oncology ward. They are with me all the way, and for that, I am so grateful.

Wednesdays with Harry
A WALK BACK IN TIME

Today we took a stroll down memory lane...

My eighty-one-year-old Dad has a heart born in Carlton, where much of it still remains. It is not only his lifelong love of AFL football and indeed the Carlton Football Club that helps his ticker beat stronger, but the familiar streets and memories of his early years.

Today, Harry and I had the delight of joining him and reliving stories and memories of those times so many years ago. Now, quite rightly, you may be thinking that this isn't Harry's cup of tea, especially when Dad turned up with a pile of maps; however, on this occasion, he appeared to look seriously interested.

We met Dad at Princes Park, the home of the Carlton Football Club, where he has been involved in recruiting since 1979 (and continues to be). As we progressed in our travels, it became clear why those with an affinity for a place also have an inherited ownership of that local footy team. They are allowed to be staunch and one-eyed. Loyalty is unquestioned, and those in their wake have wisely learnt to follow.

The highlighted line on the map indicated that we were off to locate Dad's first kindergarten. After some minor disagreements on map reading among the males in the vehicle were resolved, we finally stumbled upon the Lady Gowrie Centre, a kindergarten located on Newry Street. Dad and his parents, Bob and Jess, lived just around the corner, and these were the wartime years, and times were tough. We stopped and chatted to an elderly lady there, with whom Dad exchanged a few memories, including discussing his aversion to tripe and silverbeet that was served regularly.

We continued our journey to locate the actual house in Station Street, where he lived. Now, here it became a little confusing with new buildings and trees appearing to interfere with Dad's memory. After some time circling the area, we decided we needed to take a photo of a house, any house, which may or may not be the actual house, but would do. However, he did recall playing cricket in the laneways and kicking the football using a paper ball wrapped in elastic bands. The clarity of the memories quickly improved as we travelled closer to Princes Park. Wilson Street was next on the list, and this was Dad's home away from home as he visited his grandparents, Will and Maude Phillips. This appeared to be a 'posher' part of town, and two doors down was the home of the Andersons. Another branch of the family and owners of the Bulla Cream Company. Not close enough to actually enjoy too much cream, however. At Wilson Street, Dad was influenced by his uncles to join their love of the Carlton Football Club. Just around the corner was Princes Park, the club's home ground, which meant that Dad and his uncles were always available to watch a match. They had the ideal viewing podium by taking a ladder to the ground and perching themselves on top of the surrounding wall.

Continuing our journey, we checked out butchers' shops, lolly shops and where trenches lined the streets during the Second World War. My grandfather was a warden, instructing residents to blacken out windows and jump into a trench should the need arise.

The last stop on tour was the Melbourne Cemetery, where Will and Maude Phillips are resting. Dad was chuffed as he remembered their grave was seven trees down from the Lygon Street gate. We may have questioned his memory when it came to the house he lived in; however, we couldn't fault it now, as precisely seven trees down from the gate was indeed their final resting place. Harry declared that their headstone wasn't big enough for him. When he left this earth, he would expect nothing less than a six-foot slab of marble, decorated with every type of carving and ornate doodah that one could fit.

I asked Harry to recap what he learned today. He loved the stories and could understand why the Carlton Football Club is so important to his Pa and our family, but he declared that it was disappointing they were pretty crap right now.

'Truth isn't always friendly, Mum.'

So that was our day. Indeed, a fascinating one and well worth the tour. I highly recommend reliving memories with those who matter. So there you go…

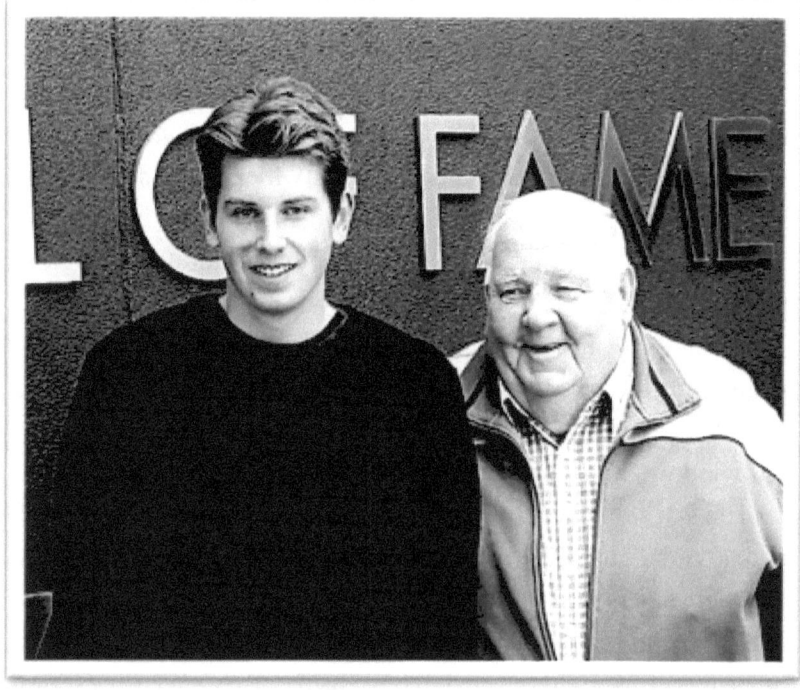

FACES OF FEAR

Many cattle stations in the Northern Territory are so isolated that the mail is flown in and supplies are trucked in weekly. If medical attention is needed, well, you either locate the first-aid box, or wait for the Flying Doctors to arrive. These properties were big, and by big, I mean millions of acres. I worked as a governess, teaching kids via the School of the Air, on one station which was three million acres.

In the early '90s, mobile phones were pretty much non-existent. Therefore, on the cattle station I was working, the only communication with the outside world at the time, was via a telephone in the manager's office or the public phone housed in the storage shed. This shed contained everything from peanut butter and baked beans to inner tyre tubes and fencing wire. The entrance had an enclosed foyer type arrangement, about 3x3 metres.

I was talking to my parents on the public phone, just on dark, when I sensed something behind me. I turned to face a King Brown, considerable size and clearly quite grumpy.

I have had quite a few encounters with its slithery cousins in my lifetime, and sorry to say, I am not a fan. In fact, I would go further and declare that I have phobic reactions of quite mammoth proportions. Therefore, you may wonder why I was working on a cattle station where Death Adders and King Browns, two of the deadliest of snakes, were known to frequent. Not sure. Anything that announces its intentions by having the word '*death*' in its name surely needs to be given a wide berth. No doubt the primary issue I have with venomous reptiles is that they can kill me, and in this current situation, I was about 700 kms from the nearest town. I was aware that a King Brown's venom could kill a cow in about twelve hours, and whilst I was not yet the size of a cow, I didn't fancy testing this theory.

I had nowhere to go. The phone was on the back wall, and my nemesis was blocking the entry. Fear rendered me petrified and frozen. I desperately hissed my situation to my parents, who were some 4000 km away in Melbourne. I am pretty sure I presented the seriousness of the circumstance quite accurately, and so, of course, there was no way my mother was going to wait until her precious one was attacked. Her very sensible solution was for me to hang up so they could call the manager and have him come and help. Brilliant idea, except for the fact that I couldn't let go of the phone. I seemed to believe that keeping them on the line would help. I was utterly paralysed, but quickly learnt that the snake had no such issues. Its quest to attack was suddenly put into motion as it reared up on its tail and was about to strike. Miraculously, at that very moment, the supply truck came hurtling into the yard. It was running three hours late due to fixing a flat and created enough reverberating racket to startle the snake, causing it to change direction, backtrack, and slither up into the arbour surrounding the entrance. I was still stuck in the shed as I didn't trust where it had gone, but my fear subsided enough to hang up and let Mum call the manager. Unloading the truck also meant jackaroos and ringers were now within cooee, so I finally used my voice and was rescued. The snake was still waiting in the arbour, but not for long - let's just say it was relocated. Much to the thirsty delight of others, the manager then unlocked a bottle of rum to remedy my quivering and trembling reaction.

Fight or flight seems to be the official term used to describe our responses to fear. I think cavemen and Sabre-Toothed Tigers are involved in the metaphor. Anyway, it is a natural, powerful, primitive human emotion that involves both biochemical and emotional reactions. Fear alerts us to danger or threat, whether physical or psychological. Sometimes it can stem from real threats, but it can also originate from imagined dangers. We prepare ourselves to either ready ourselves for combat or run away. In this case, I certainly wasn't prepared for battle and would have happily run away if that option were available. I managed to experience both physical and mental reactions. It is all about survival. I believe fear saved me that night. It alerted me to the danger and kept me from any sudden movements. There are a lot of fancy words connected to this, but the nutshell is that fear can be helpful; it can save our arses from danger, but I have also discovered that when it comes to having an incurable disease, fear can also be the enemy.

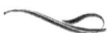

Looking back on a favoured and memorable decade, I would absolutely declare that the ten-year period from the mid'80s was mine. Not at all surprising that these halcyon days were when I was in my twenties. I was travelling the world, seeking adventures. I loved every minute, from aimlessly backpacking around Europe to being employed as a nanny in the UK and northern Italy. Working for Contiki Tours in Europe and New Zealand, and finally sweltering on cattle stations and tourist resorts in Australia's outback.

For my generation, these '80s/'90s glory days meant we had yet to discover; healthy eating, responsible recycling, dental perfection, Wikipedia, hair straighteners, Google, gluten intolerance, mobile phones, social media, fake news, global warming, drinking in moderation, terrorism, manscaping, ozone issues, bitcoin, digital everything, and that every kiddy received a prize. We worked hard and played hard. Life was to be lived, and the music was brilliant. We danced the night away to AC/DC, INXS and U2. Springsteen screamed he was born in the USA, and Queen declared that fat-bottomed girls made the rocking world go round. It was one of the most extravagant decades in cultural history.

For all that I loved about this era, it was also a time that was one of the most tragic eras in terms of health. The AIDS epidemic. It began as a predominantly African disease, followed by being associated with the gay community.

In 1985, it was announced that Rock Hudson had died from complications of AIDS. The fact that he was gay was not the shock. It was the idea that AIDS could affect even the rich and famous. The Western world sat up and took notice. The fear of AIDS/HIV became real. It was also hideously riddled with shame and guilt, with the onus being placed on the gay profile.

In 1989, I worked in publicity at the State Film Centre of Victoria, and I was required to distribute condoms at the Gay Film Festival. The suggestion and association to AIDS were absolutely in your face, and whilst it was supposedly a sign of the times, I, for one, objected to handing out such latex judgements.

HIV continues to be a significant global health issue. The World Health Organisation estimates that some thirty-six million lives have been lost so far. At the end of 2020, approximately thirty-seven million people were living with HIV, with two-thirds from African regions. There are still too many deaths and no cure. Thankfully, access to prevention, early diagnosis and treatment has meant it becomes a more manageable chronic health condition, enabling many people with AIDS to live long and healthy lives.

The fear of AIDS changed the rules regarding safe sex, sharing syringes, transfusions, blood rules on sporting fields, etc., culminating in awareness for us all.

Fear has been used as a marketing strategy for some time. Its roots go back to the 1920s when Listerine created a mouthwash to tackle halitosis. The original ad campaign centred on a young woman struggling to find someone to marry because of her stinky breath. The slogan read, 'Halitosis makes you unpopular!'

One of the most infamous and criticised scaremongering advertising campaigns of our time was the Grim Reaper commercials shown in the late 80s as a deterrent for AIDS. They were shockingly graphic and had the sole aim of projecting fear into the broader community. I remember them well, and as far as creating terror and phobia, they did their job. Until recently, I hadn't thought about that campaign for over thirty years. I was attempting to explain why I feel it is so important to try and defuse the fear that comes with a cancer diagnosis and how debilitating anxiety can be, and the AIDS Grim Reaper ads popped into my mind. I viewed those ads as a scare campaign to create a reaction, but at no time did it occur to me how it would feel to watch such propaganda if you already had AIDS. I now get it.

The interpretation of such an ad would be very different if you were already suffering from AIDS. Would you be able to fend off such imagery, or would you be consumed with an undeniable fear? Terminal illness is seen as hopeless, but I can assure you, hope is the one thing you cling to regardless. The Grim Reaper ensures that all hope is lost.

It seems to me that there is a fine line between deliberately using fear to promote action and where fear can become overwhelming and leave you paralysed. Its use may encourage knowledge and education, early detection and even fundraising, but what if you already have a terminal diagnosis? Believing I will die a horrid and painful death from cancer may be seen as the truth, but is that thought actually helpful to my own quality and length of life? In some Asian countries, for example, China and Japan, until recently, any advanced cancer diagnosis was only disclosed to the family. The patient would be denied that knowledge with the thought that they would be so stressed that their body wouldn't cope and certainly wouldn't heal. They connected damaging physical responses to psychological emotions and concluded that ignorance is bliss.

Whilst I have elected to be knowledgeably informed and realise I need to face my fears, I also understand how fear can creep up and instigate a physical ill effect alongside the emotional reaction of hopelessness. This topic reaches into the unknown. Difficult to scientifically test how powerful our minds are and whether physical effects can be altered by thought. I think it is incredibly fascinating and creates so many questions. Why are placebos effective? So many questions...

Cancer seems to thrive on fear. While fear can be helpful to get you out of your seat, take action to seek medical attention and advance your health, it can also keep you terrified and result in an unhealthy and debilitating emotion. If allowed, it can stifle your choices and strangle your freedom. Many times, it roars, many times it niggles, and many times is not relevant or necessary.

I don't often talk about fear; however, my way of dealing with it is to understand that thoughts cannot hurt me and to try to stay present...And to also avoid venomous reptiles in outback sheds!

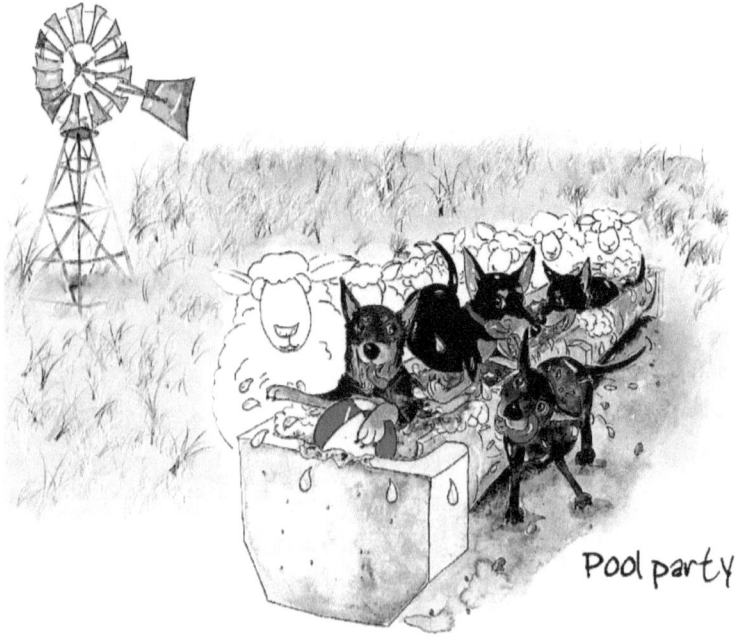

Pool party

Wednesdays with Harry
RONE EMPIRE

I had acquired two of the now sold-out tickets to the Rone Empire exhibit at Burnham Beeches in the Dandenongs. Rone is the name of the artist, known for his exceptional street art skills. Burnham Beeches is a magnificent Art Deco mansion that has been vacant for approximately twenty years. Before renovations were to begin restoring it to its previous glory, for the past year, Rone had taken over and applied his artist's imaginings to the entire house. Every room has been transported into a bygone era, filled with Art Deco furniture and memories, autumn leaves and branches, cobwebs, and dust, all accompanied by the artist's impression of his muse, Lily Sullivan.

It is indeed The Great Gatsby meets Funny Farm and the Addams Family. You feel you have intruded on the past, yet eerily, the past has left in a hurry. Throughout the dilapidated, decaying, ramshackle building, it is easy to imagine the glory days; sipping cocktails on the south lawn, Billie Holiday teasing the mood and where life was simple and carefree.

I was pleasantly surprised at Harry's interest in the exhibit, although he questioned the need for so many twigs and leaves filling old chairs and corners.

The outlined rules of admission were brief, but they did include not touching anything in the exhibit. I reminded Harry of this on several occasions, when he felt that he could perhaps add his own creative rearrangement. And...inevitably, he just couldn't seem to help himself, and so the pool table now shows evidence of a dust-free circle where once a snooker ball was artistically placed.

With its watery floor, the library, where leather chairs and bookshelves are semi-submerged in the blue pool, was a favourite. Every room reflected the past, and with artificial flowers, Art Deco pipe stands, and heavy velvet curtains, the memory of Grandparents fondly reminisced.

In the final part of the exhibit, you are invited to watch a short film on the making of the installation by wearing virtual reality goggle thingies. Suddenly, my world was filled with the entire project 360 degrees and viewed from my rotating chair.

Now it may be that the giddiness I have been experiencing lately was partly to blame, but my medication was no match for this virtual reality experience. It spun me right off my chair, and just in case I wasn't embarrassed enough, the attendant removed the goggle thingies and caught them in the clasps holding on my 'hair'.

I swayed and staggered my way to the exit, woozy head in one hand and skewwhiff hair in the other.

So there you go…

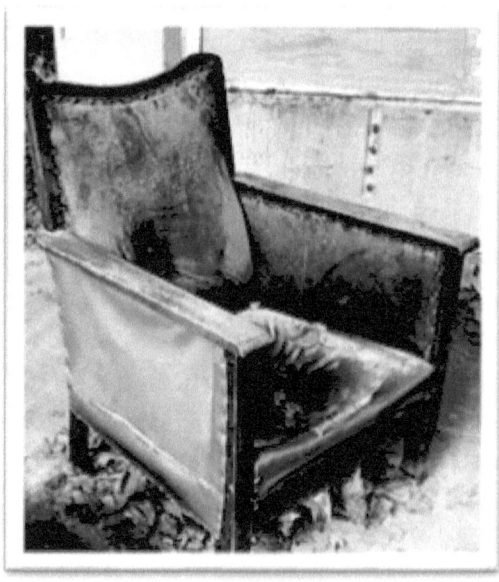

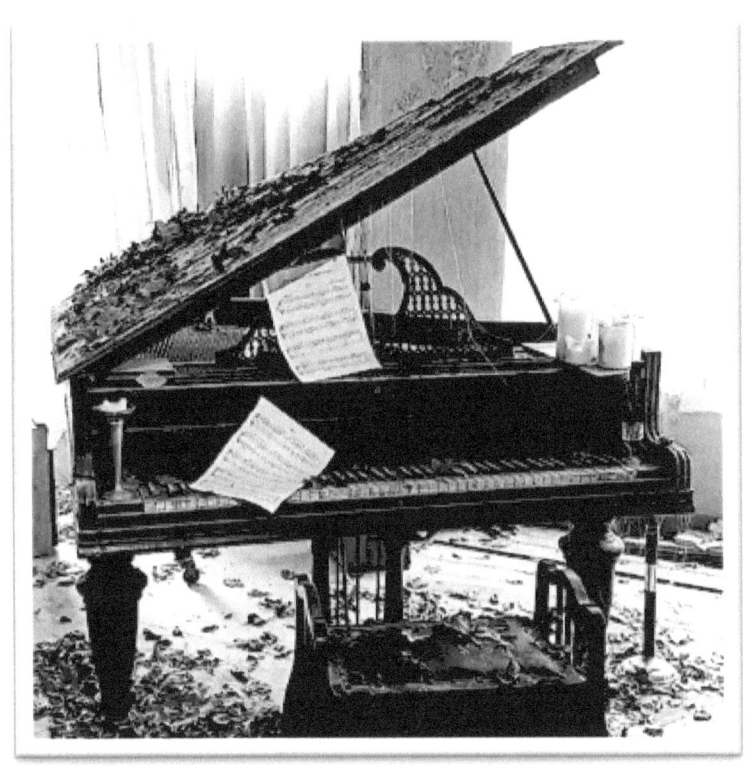
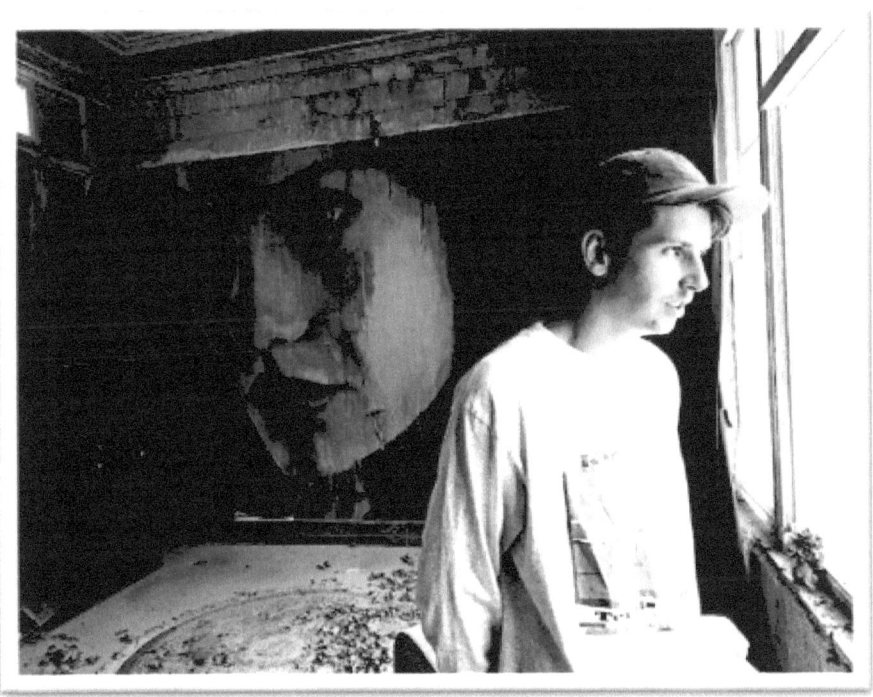

CASUALTY OF CANCER

If you have miraculously made it thus far, then hopefully, you may have concluded that I am being as straight up and candid as possible. I am exposed. At the very least, this account needs to come from my heart.

I met Bryce while working at El Questro Station Wilderness Park, a tourist resort located in the Kimberley region of Western Australia. It was in the early '90s and when El Questro, initially a cattle station, was in the beginning stages of poking its toe in the tourism waters. A million acres of the most rugged yet fragile and serene landscape I have known. It was undoubtedly the most fantastic adventure that has had such a profound influence on my life. The people I met there are still some of my closest friends. That tends to happen when you are united in unique and extraordinary situations. Any challenges that arose from working in such a remote destination were totally insignificant compared to the fulfilment and gratitude I felt from my experiences.

Bryce and I married during our time there in 1994, and now, 27 years later, in 2022, as this book goes to print, we are experiencing the sadness and finality of divorce.

It isn't bitter; there isn't anger or blame, just the realisation that it's time for honesty and to agree that we should no longer be husband and wife. For quite some time, we had both fallen into an incurious and dormant version of what a marriage should be. So many elements were mislaid. Choosing to end something so familiar was hard, but living a life that is not true is not really living.

I have often wondered if having cancer delayed or influenced this decision. We have both acknowledged that our marriage was drifting apart before my diagnosis. No matter how challenging or complex the cancer rollercoaster is, finding a solution can be impossible if the fundamentals are missing.

Sometimes adversity creates unity, a lasting bond, and closeness—and sometimes it creates division.

Everyone has different ways and levels of coping. In this case, expectations and support eventually became too hard.

There is a feeling of stepping out on a ledge without a safety net, and whilst filled with sadness and grief, it comes as a reminder that having cancer is no excuse to remain stagnant. I am happy for Bryce to find whatever he needs for a fulfilling future.

Finality is quite a powerful word, and I am feeling its weight right now. The knowledge that I will never again be in a relationship is difficult to reconcile. Choice and inevitability are two separate ideals that will eventually merge into acceptance.

I look forward to that day.

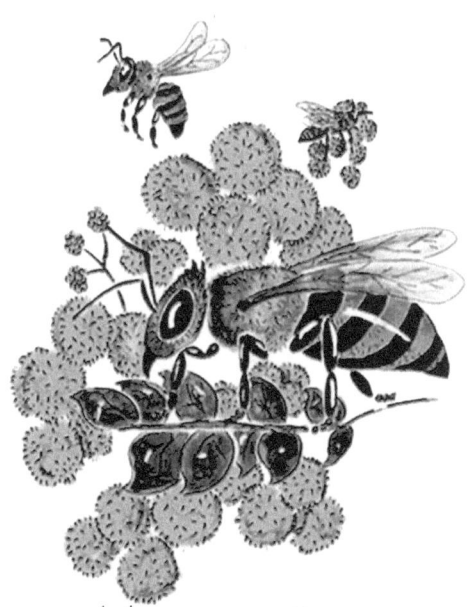

wattle bee will bee

Wednesdays with Harry
STREET SOUNDS

A short but satisfying outing saw us strolling along the posh South Yarra streets, majestically lined with historic homes, wrought-iron fences and knobbly trees. For some reason, Jane Austin terminology 'take a turn' springs to mind as our sole purpose is to observe and meander with a pleasant tête-à-tête mid amble. Now, when I say 'we', that is, of course, me. Whilst my mind was firmly fixed in the Regency era with high expectations of gentle sophistication, the reality of wearing a bum bag and leopard-skin Crocs absolutely shatters this illusion. On the other hand, Harry is never content with a stroll and once again believes it is his mission to keep me moving as quickly as possible.

There is always a point in these leisurely walks at which Harry's patience is tested. I attempt to amuse him with my light-hearted conversation, hoping he will be distracted and oblivious to the pace. However, my speed slowed even further as I paused to take snapshots of ironwork and tree roots. Harry's opposition to my photo indulgence is clear. The usual pattern commences. He seems to assume that the more he insults my sensibilities, the more I will suddenly put the camera aside and break into a sprint. Never test a mother who has a point to prove, or in fact, is too unfit to go any quicker. Taking the high road and continuing my lively chatter, we finally reach that juncture. That point in the conversation when Harry is holding on tight to remain stern, grim and serious. But the crack slowly appears. He hates it when he tries to stay cross, yet a wave of wit has him break into a grin. Aha – my jesting triumphs again. Humour is my mediator, my rescue remedy, my hero and saviour!

We continue to stroll. It is early evening, and workers are heading home, diners are spilling to the outside cafes, and joggers are sweating their socks off. Now speaking of socks, one such jogger wore knee-high socks. Harry explained that he was wearing compression socks, which were supposed to help prevent lactic acid from building up. I briefly confused this with lactose intolerance and wondered how socks could possibly help with a bloated gut. Fortunately, I kept that thought to myself whilst my brain quickly adjusted and realised the difference. I then asked Harry if he would rather have lactic acid build-up or run in those socks.

'Wouldn't ever choose to look like a knob, Mum', he stated.

So, we strolled on back, perilously dodging the numerous phone addicted zombies that recklessly roamed the streets. They stride along, oblivious to surroundings, oncoming traffic, fellow androids and dog poo.

So there you go…

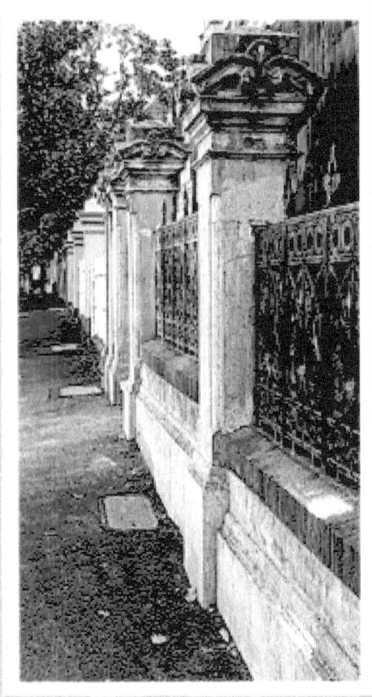

FAMILY

I have often felt guilty regarding the weight of cancer and its effect on my family. I feel that where once untroubled and light-hearted moments may have dominated family gatherings, in more recent times, my illness has contributed to more sombre attitudes. We just don't seem to laugh as loud or as often as we did. So, I absolutely recognise that my situation has affected those close by. They have their own emotions, thoughts and demons that need to be noticed. I have invited my family to include some notes about their own emotions, thoughts and feelings and here are responses from my sisters, parents, Bryce and Harry.

I vividly remember the day you were first told that you had breast cancer. I got the shakes and left work in tears to meet you at Mum and Dad's. It shook me. There have been times that I have worried about asking you how things are going for fear that things weren't great. I have also had thoughts of how amazing you have handled all this (on the outside). You have shown such amazing courage and have always had such a positive outlook. I would say that I have cried, laughed and worried about you over the years. You are so strong, and I feel like I haven't always understood how you are really feeling.

Through all of this, I love that you have always put Harry first, and he is one amazing young man. You have toughed this out mostly on your own, which I suppose I have taken for granted.

You are the most amazing, wonderful sister, who I am so very proud of all your achievements in health, business and life. Love you, Lynne xx

---

I have been giving this some thought, and whilst I think every emotion has come into play at some stage over your cancer journey, the one that stands out the most is a pure sense of helplessness.

When you told us in 2011 you had breast cancer, the sense of not knowing what to do or say was ever-present. I took Mum to Donvale rehab and told Dad you had cancer; as he cried, I realised that the impact of this news was huge; not only did I not know how to help you, I didn't know how to make Mum and Dad feel better either.

Watching you suffer through the chemo and its side effects will remain with me forever. On occasion, I came to Warburton to see you inconsolable with fear, not for yourself, but for Harry. Not knowing what to say, trying to stay strong, then crying on the way home again with a sense of helplessness. I remember trying to get you organised as you struggled with a container of various drugs, not knowing which ones to take when chemo brain had set in.

The operation to remove your breast was so painful for you, and so was the radiation therapy, but again, I couldn't take it away. Worrying about not only your health but everything that goes with it. How were you going to go emotionally, financially, and physically?

We could help from a distance but couldn't take away the pain or worry you were experiencing. I could go to treatment with you and learn a little about the process, but I would never totally understand what you were experiencing. The side effects were at times worse as we watched you lose your hair, experience brittle nails and the ongoing neuropathy, and lymphedema, which has only continued to get worse. Again, things that we could not totally understand.

You gained a great deal of strength over time, and you were incredibly determined. It was inspiring to see the inner strength you demonstrated. There were also times of genuine frustration with doctors who seemed to be messing you around. Additionally, I feel frustrated that you wouldn't allow us to accompany you to appointments. Over time, I realised that this was your journey, and you were going to do it your way; it did not matter what I thought should happen, as it was about what you needed to do to get through as best as possible. There were times when we investigated alternative therapy, such as the Gawler Foundation in Yarra Junction, and tried to find some cannabis oil to help, anything that might help.

In 2015, the terminal diagnosis was so hard to witness. I waited outside for you at your appointment, praying everything would be okay. As you approached me, the look on your face told me the news wasn't good, and the heartache you experienced again brought back that overwhelming sense of helplessness. How do we help? How do we take this away for you? How do you go through new treatment plans, pain both physically and emotionally? New treatment started, and I learnt a little by coming along to treatment and watching the nurse struggling to access your port. I admired how you kept your spirits up every three weeks. The bond you formed with the oncology nurses was great to see, and I know this continues. It took me a while to adjust to not being able to come during Covid, as it was just a little thing to do to help feel like I was supporting you in some way. Other hospital visits were also frustrating. We waited for several hours at times, just to see a doctor, only to be told to go to another department to get access to your stupid port, knowing that you just wanted to get out of there. Still, again, I couldn't do anything to help except sit there and try to distract you somehow. This was only a few times, so I can only imagine the frustration you feel as you wait endlessly for appointments. I hate to think how many hours you've spent in waiting rooms over the years!

Each time you go for scans, we hold our breath and hope for good news, again only from a distance, and cannot imagine how you get through the waiting. Your inner strength grew with time; thanks to the knowledge that treatment was keeping things at bay. Your sense of humour, creativity, and drive have returned. You got on with your life supporting Harry wholeheartedly, which was, I think, your primary drive over this journey. In some ways, it is like you are each other's rocks in life.

With your diagnosis, we have been screened. It has allowed us to get advice and hopefully safeguard ourselves from breast cancer, and let our daughters take steps to protect themselves. As I said at the start, your cancer journey has undoubtedly been a rollercoaster of emotions, but nothing, of course, close to what you personally have experienced.

I truly admire how you have handled this journey with grit, humour, dignity, and grace. As your journey continues, I hope that we can help in any way, even if it means an overall sense of helplessness.

Love Gai xx

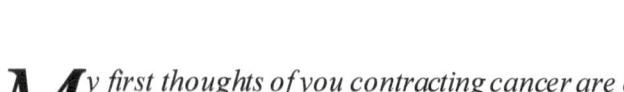

My first thoughts of you contracting cancer are clearly stuck in my head. I was in Donvale doing rehab when Mum and Gai came in and told me. I did not sleep that night, wondering how and why. Were you too close to Chernobyl?

I wanted to be home with Jean to see how we could help. I was angry that you were in this situation and wanted to protect you. Then, four years later, you told us the cancer had spread and was now incurable and that you possibly only had a few years to live. Again, we felt helpless. I prayed every night. Maybe that helped me realise your strength to fight with every bit of knowledge you could gather to beat this beast.

Your attitude to bringing up Harry through all this has been, to me, your greatest ally.

The number of treatments and drugs you have endured has been incredible. You have shown us courage and bravery beyond the call and are still dealing with it.

We wish and hope that the beast will go away for good.

Love, Dad xx

*L*ooking back over the years of your trial of having cancer, it mostly makes me feel useless to help you either practically or financially. You have certainly been through so much, but your determination and courage have been outstanding.

We have offered many times to help by going with you to the hospital, but you have preferred to do it your way. We then get very annoyed at circumstances such as you wanting to drive yourself and having to park a mile away – why can't the hospital give you a parking area close to where you have treatment? Why can't they lessen the time you spend waiting for an appointment? Would things be any better if you had private health cover?

The nurses involved with your treatment have certainly been very supportive, and I am sure you have formed quite a few friendships there.

You have had a couple of close friends support you with love and humour, so we are grateful for their help.

I think the medical treatment has caused so much harm with radiation burns etc. – surely there must be a better way! Frustration comes all the time when we cannot change the circumstances.

Why did you get cancer? – Was it your time overseas near Chernobyl, or were you just unlucky? Love Mum xx

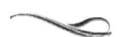

Jo's journey through cancer has been since 2011, and of course, we have all been intertwined throughout this. Reading this book, you will understand the various stages of cancer and some of the side effects of treatment she has endured, and you will be right in thinking that it has been a horrific journey. But even though at times cancer has dominated parts of her life, she still lives life. She has not stopped being Jo.

Although she comes across as putting cancer on the back burner, I think she always has had it in her mind the actual situation she is in and the real prospects that could occur. She has tackled pretty much all of it on her own, making her a strong and brave woman. She has had support from family, but really had to deal with the demons on her own. Then, where were you, I hear you ask? Did I or have I offered enough support to Jo over the years? The short answer is no, I haven't, and I'm not sure why. I never seemed to know the right words to say when she was suffering.

At a men's gathering once for partners of cancer sufferers, most there discussed that they went to every appointment and treatment with their partner. I really didn't go to many. Generally, I felt she preferred I didn't, but did I know that for sure? If I could go back in time, perhaps...

I heard that if your marriage is not strong enough to begin with, then this challenging journey may well lead to an end. And yes, after twenty-seven years, our marriage has concluded. I'm definitely not blaming Jo's cancer, as we had begun drifting apart at some point before her diagnosis, but it definitely added plenty more pressure and stress. Some couples thrive and become closer, and some don't.

Harry and I seem to be two males who are not necessarily insensitive but find it challenging to appear sympathetic and say all the right things. There were times when Jo was travelling along okay, and we probably just got on with life and wouldn't give her situation enough thought. When she needed more treatment or became ill, it was a solid reminder that life is not that simple.

After every setback, Jo seemingly bounces back to her busy, incredible self, and it has really been something to admire and be proud of. She still takes on everything with the same vigour, and although she has regular treatment for stage IV cancer and suffers the ups and downs, she is still Jo. Cancer has never owned her.

So, how do I feel overall about Jo having cancer and its effect on family life? I am slow at adapting and evolving, and will always regret not being naturally supportive enough, not being communicative enough, and not being proactive enough to tackle all that is involved with a cancer diagnosis. However, despite our marriage coming to an end, I still look forward to being part of her life, and we will always share our history together. Her commitment to everything she does is remarkable, even writing this book. Bryce

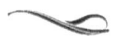

I can't remember too much when Mum was first diagnosed. I do recollect Mum breaking the news to me; however, I was eleven, so pretty young at the time. At first, I didn't know how to feel or grasp what was happening to the full extent. Being exposed to what Mum

was going through at a young age was probably a good thing in a sense.

The next time she had to go through chemo, I started to comprehend the full magnitude of what was happening. A significant moment in gaining this understanding was when Mum began to lose her hair because that was a visual symbol of cancer. I was worried and concerned about what was happening and what could happen in the future.

I am not a very sentimental person, but I am told that there were times when I was emotional about Mum. My recollection of this is somewhat faded; perhaps that's a subconscious decision I made. Whilst Mum's situation is challenging, she has made it much easier than I imagined it would and could be. It's surprising when you consider what has happened. Mum's cancer is not often at the forefront of thought. Life has continued mostly as usual because Mum has created that perception; hence her term 'chasing normal'. How she has dealt with her circumstance, I believe, has helped not only the people around her but also Mum. I really admire how she has handled what she has been dealt with.

Love you, Mum. Harry xx

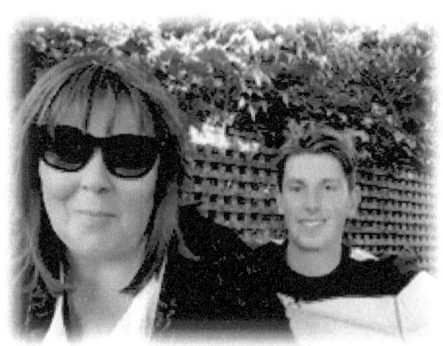

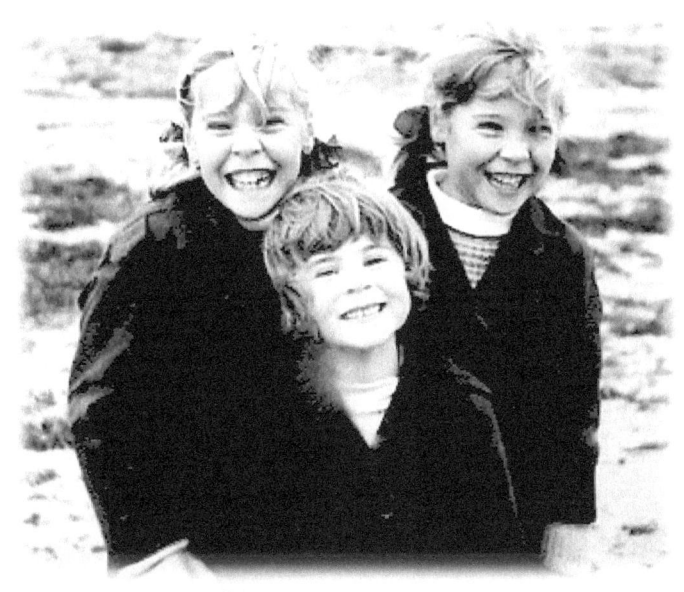

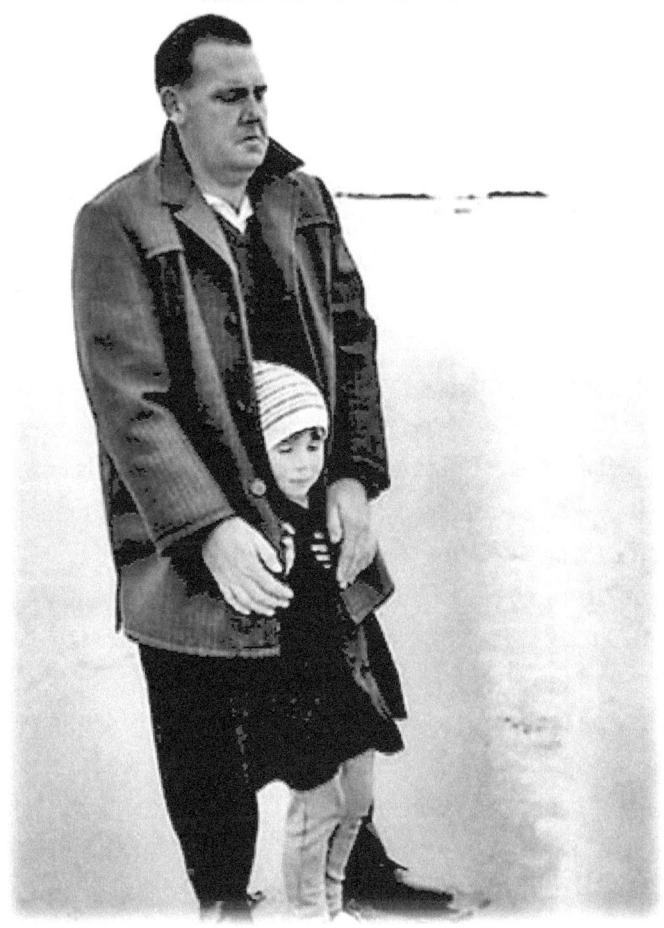

Wednesdays with Harry
BOLLARDS

My feet are sore, my bones are stiff, my body is inflamed, and I believe cramp is not far away. This is the aftermath of meeting the challenge.

Today, we decided to venture to Geelong and walk the Bollard Trail. In keeping with the maritime theme, the foreshore of Geelong features bollards that have been expertly carved and painted into a fantastic array of whimsical sculptures. I briefly read the blurb, and whilst I realised there were forty-eight bollards to sight, I scoffed at the suggestion it would take us two hours to walk it. That must be a typo, I thought. We began the trail a little late in the day, but not a problem, we would do a quick tour, grab some lunch and be back on the road before the peak hour traffic hit. I checked out the map, and it did appear that they had stretched these bollards out quite a distance. So from Matthew Flinders to Life Saving Clubs, to Bathing Beauties, Peter Lalor, Salvation Army Woman, Nancy Nattyknickers and Nuns and countless others were on parade awaiting our visit. When 3:30 pm ticked over, the question was raised whether anyone would actually care, or in fact, know, if we finished this task. Argh! Those morality lessons in life that a parent must impart to their child. Of course, we had to finish.

Plodding along the Bob McGavan Memorial Path, I realised that many of these bollards would only likely be seen by joggers, dog walkers and those few foolish nutters that loved a challenge. So, avoiding the odd dog doo-doo, goobers from sweaty spitting joggers and ducks on the attack, we finally reached the end; that is, we reached number forty-seven bollard. Okay, this cannot be. Where is forty-eight? After more searching, by now on crumbling legs (mine), we sat down for a think. I reread the list and finally found the fine print that bollard forty-eight, Morris Jacobs from Jacobs stores, had been relocated to the Carousel. Of course, he was. Harry's gizmo on his watch clocked our journey at 7.45 km. So whilst I was somewhat humbled that I scoffed at the two-hour suggestion, I was more concerned that I was able to crawl back to the car without total collapse.

You will be pleased to know that we made it back and sank into the comfort of the car. Harry then had a swig of water, and as he held up his bottle to drink, a soft jelly lolly came fluttering down from above. Perplexity was eventually met with clarity as I realised that it must have attached itself to the underside of his bottle and flown through the air when tipped upward. This small and insignificant moment suddenly triggered a flashback to a memory of a similar, yet far more impactful, mystery that occurred many years ago when I was in high school.

I had arrived at school and put my bag on the nature strip for a minute. I picked it up and walked into school, totally oblivious that I had put my bag on dog poo which in turn had attached itself to the bottom of my bag. I put my bag on top of my locker, not sure how, but still blissfully unaware. I then noticed an odour - it was coming from the side of my strides, and I was shocked and appalled to discover it was poo. Just like Harry's lolly, although far more devastating, I had no idea how poo had landed on my leg! My mind was exploding with outrageous confusion and mayhem. I headed to the toilets, scrubbed my strides, and then continued to art class, still baffled and horrified and massively concerned that my peers may detect my stinky poo pants. Upon returning to my locker, I realised the offensive stench was overwhelming, and upon further investigation, I finally understood what had happened.

With other bags jostling for position, the poo had now spread like icing on a cake across the top of the lockers, and of course, I had the pleasant task of spending recess cleaning the mess.

Safe to say, I have not placed my bag on the ground since, without a full field reconnaissance and a completed scientific soil survey.

So there you go...

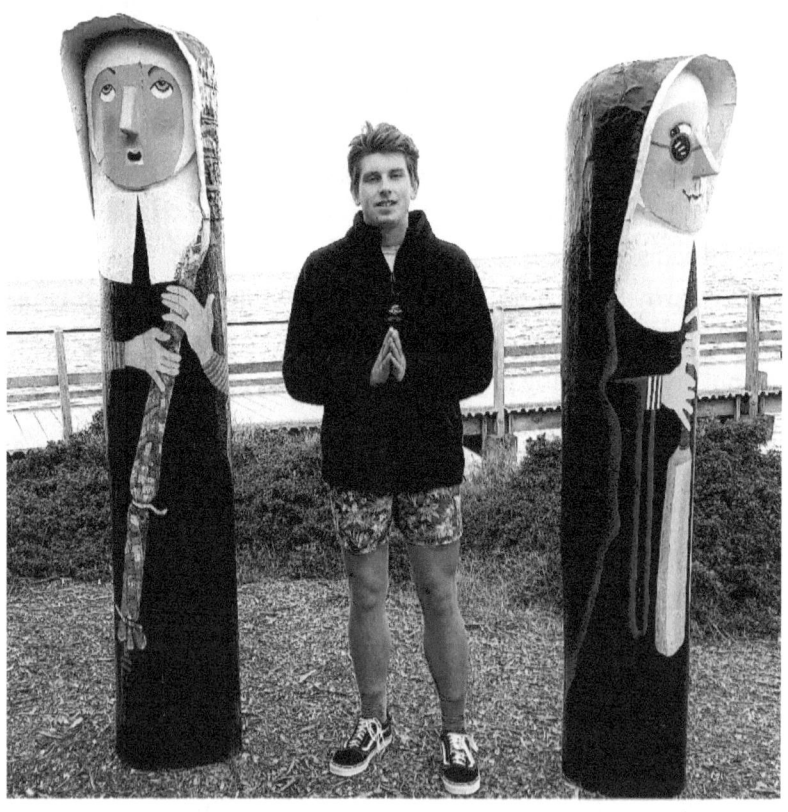

PAIN PARANOIA

May, 2022

Some years ago, I recalled Stephen Fry declaring that there was no such thing as pain. His explanation followed the failed attempts from panellists on the television program *QI* to reply with accuracy. Stephen Fry's intellect is undoubtedly above average and should never be questioned, but how can pain actually not exist? Well, apparently, pain is constructed entirely in the brain. Your brain creates what your body feels, and therefore, pain is simply perceived. Feeling pain is our brain relaying a message. Anyone who has pushed out a 4.5 kg child without any medical assistance may offer a different insight!

As I am writing this, I have an ache in my left upper arm. It has been there for a few weeks; I question its origin and have become a little paranoid. Anyone who knows cancer also knows that it can crop up anywhere in the body and present as pain. My apprehension simply reinforces the notion that, despite my fierce declaration of how pointless and unhelpful paranoia is, I am still capable of being seduced into its web.

The paranoia process begins moderately quietly as I logically try to ascertain where I could have strained my upper arm muscle. Could it be from when I reached up to change the clock battery? Not really straining there, perhaps it was from carrying a heavy bag of shopping? I have a vague notion that I may have done that - or did I? I desperately cling to any distant idea that may validate this pain. The paranoia grows. It hurts when I am just sitting still. Should that happen? And now it's starting to itch; what's that all about? I fight the urge to search on the internet. I win that particular battle, but the niggling concern remains and begins to snowball.

I have regular CT scans, usually about every three to four months, and every second one includes a bone scan. I now think that we missed the last bone scan – now, when was that? More than eight months ago? Paranoia continues to escalate.

One of my personality traits appears to be that I remain fairly restrained in my responses to situations where others may show excitement. It is not that I don't feel enthused; I just don't tend to animate my reactions. Harry definitely has developed the same trait. I need further reasoning and validation for this particular pain, so bring Harry into the conversation. He is pursuing a degree in Sports Science, and therefore studies muscles, among other things.

His answer is completely lacking in concern as he explains that someone as unfit and old as I could easily pull a muscle by simply getting out of bed. He also reminds me of all the other times I have gone through such pains—the tennis elbow, the left hip bursitis, the right hip bursitis, the gallstone, the bible cyst, the backache, the shoulder pain, the pancreatic infection—and they turned out to be precisely what they were supposed to be.

Harry is unaware that his complacent response, although ageist and somewhat unsympathetic, is precisely what I needed to quell my apprehension. He is correct; I have worried myself over aches and pains in the past that have turned out to be nothing out of the ordinary.

Will this paranoia ever truly subside? Or, for that matter, my own contradictions? I blab on that a thought cannot hurt me, yet here I am again, tangled up in notions, ideas and beliefs that are messing with my mind.

Oh, and Harry also reminded me that there is no such thing as pain…

Wednesdays with Harry
MAGICAL MYSTERY TOUR

After my suggestion to enjoy a free preview performance of The Wizard of Oz was met with a very rude rebuttal, I decided to change tack and go for a drive instead. We would follow our own yellow brick road, so our day was now going to be 'The Magical Mystery Tour.'

I wrote the words 'Left,' 'Right,' and 'Straight' on several cards and put them in a bag. Today's rule was that Harry randomly picked a card at every major intersection, which, in turn, determined the direction we took. Any time an option was, in fact, not an option, he had to choose again. When 1 p.m. ticked over, the tour would end, and we would stop for lunch at the closest town.

Harry declared that it was a crazy idea and that we were likely to end up driving in circles, completely wasting his time and that this tour was not at all magical. He did, however, agree to give it a go.

Following the cards, we were led to Melbourne and over the Westgate Bridge. Unfortunately, the roads that followed were indeed leading us around in circles for some time after that.

At the beginning of this journey, I did imagine that it would be lovely if we happened to venture to the picturesque town of Mount Macedon or perhaps enjoy a leisurely lunch of calamari somewhere along the bay. Alas, we seemed to be stuck in a spiralling labyrinth of asphalt at the arse end of the earth, and lunch was looking like sharing a sausage roll with a bloke called Bluey, sold from the back of a van. Sorry to offend anyone who resides or treasures places such as Laverton, Altona or Point Cook.

At one point, I caught Harry googling a map and suspect he may have manipulated a couple of instruction cards to get us out of there.

Finally, we ended up on the highway to Geelong, and with few options but straight ahead, we had time for a chat. The topic of Mother's Day came up. Harry is quite reluctant on most occasions to open his wallet, so when he inquired about what I would like as a gift, I was a little surprised. I explained that I didn't need him to purchase a gift. I did, however, suggest that he give me what I ask for every Birthday, Mother's Day and Christmas, and that is that the windows are washed, the bathroom scrubbed, and the floors cleaned. (Yet to happen, by the way.) He emphatically declared that he would rather buy me a twenty-dollar bottle of perfume. He then indignantly, yet genuinely, inquired why, in fact, there is no Son's Day. I have no words!

Besides a quick detour past the North Shore refinery, we managed to eventually make our way to the other side of Geelong, twenty-five minutes before the tour was to end. Finally, the cards played in our favour, and we ended up in the gorgeous town of Portarlington.

Sitting outside with sea views and eating our chicken salad roll at the most fabulous bakery was a joy and definitely worth the trip.

So there you go...

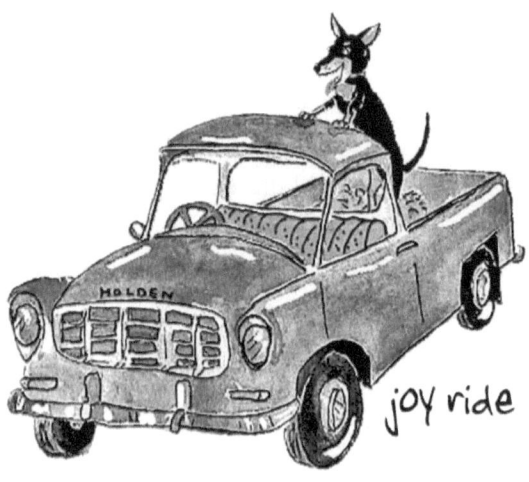

joy ride

RIDING HIGH IN APRIL, SHOT DOWN IN MAY

May, 2022

The pain in my arm that I mentioned was still there and becoming more constant and severe.

As I was in between oncology appointments, I went to my GP to investigate. I was sent for an ultrasound and an X-ray. He called the following day with the results and explained that the X-ray showed a lesion, an erosion in my humerus. I sucked in briefly and asked the question. That question that you ask but don't really want to hear the answer to. Remaining in ignorance is definitely a blissful state to be in. Life can continue without intrusion; however, you may eventually pay the price. So, grasping at all the straws on the planet, I asked, *'Is there anything other than cancer that would cause a lytic lesion in my bone?'* I felt physically sick when he replied that he couldn't tell me there was.

The follow-up tests were a bone scan and a CT scan, organised for the following Monday. The incredibly kind receptionist at radiology understood the urgency and ensured I could be seen as soon as possible. So, I had five days to get through before tests would confirm if cancer was up and about and creating more havoc.

To be honest, I feel like such a fraud. I prattle on about taking away the power of cancer, staying present, and that fear is just imagining the future. Yet, my initial reaction was the absolute epitome of someone being swallowed in a sea of fear and dread. So many thoughts were galloping around in my mind, and they all signalled gloom. I do, however, feel grateful that I have completed plenty of work on my mental health in the past, so it was time to put it into practice. Distraction and diffusion do work for at least part of the time.

I managed to occupy myself during the days, but the stampede of thoughts trampled my mind when the night came. They needed to be collected, expressed and unloaded. Late at night, when the quiet creeps in, I wait for actuality to be acknowledged. Sleep didn't happen. Exhaustion running alongside trepidation creates an emotional train wreck. I have come to understand there is a process involved in grieving one's health issues. The initial reaction is a torrid downpour that lasts a couple of days or until I regroup and calm my mind. Once I can reinstate some rationality, I look for answers that I already know I have. The most significant thought that whacks me fair square in the noggin is:

If I truly have faith that I will not die from cancer, then what do I have to fear?

The can of worms is opened when someone with advanced cancer has an apparently naïve notion that they, in fact, will live and deny the terminal prognosis. The medical fraternity will look upon such an idea with gentle sympathy for one in such denial, and no doubt, they regularly encounter the heartbreaking use of hope. Terms such as *false hope* are mentioned. By the way, there is no such thing as *false hope*. Hope is hope. But I am not just talking about hope; I am talking about faith—a true belief that cannot be broken. Having felt the eruption of fear this last week clearly states that I am not there yet.

I have a book called *Radical Remissions* that I gravitate towards in such times as these. The author, Kelly A. Turner, travelled the globe seeking out cancer patients who, for whatever reason, had survived their medically advanced cancer prognosis and are now cancer-free. She researched the common factors that these people had and compiled her findings and case studies. Many of the similar aspects were regarding our mental attitude. Now, this isn't about just 'thinking positively'. It is so much more, and it is a subject that sparks numerous opinions and debates. I have no doubt you may have the most positive attitude in existence, and still may die from cancer. No one would accept that someone died from cancer because they didn't have the faith not to. Without scientific support for such a phenomenon, however, it will continue to be debated and questioned, leaving a definitive answer elusive. Our physical and mental health is a combination of individuality, and so what I think, feel, or respond to is entirely my own. Comparisons to others who have died from cancer or those who haven't are quite irrelevant. In times of stress, panic and anxiety, however, the knowledge that those still existing with terminal cancer is helpful. What is real is yours alone.

One of the case studies in this book was about a Japanese bloke who was sent home with no further medical intervention able to help him. Among the various outlooks he practised was to love his cancer. He couldn't understand why being angry at something that was part of him would be helpful, so he decided to nurture it. This resonated with me.

You may have noticed that at the beginning of this book, I speak about cancer as a beast that I needed to rid my body of, no matter what. Over the years, I have come to understand that these cells are part of me, and whilst they are dangerously rebellious and need some stern encouragement to behave, hating them simply causes me unnecessary grief.

Monday morning arrived, and for whatever reason, I suddenly calmed down. The process at the hospital radiology department was well-rehearsed. I am very familiar with the procedures, and the feeling of calm allowed my mind to start visualising a cancer-free body. I do this regularly when I have scans. I have a mental picture of my internal bits without cancer and concentrate on that image during scanning.

The CT scans were first up. I always recognise many staff members, but I understand that it is unlikely they will remember me, given the thousands of patients they constantly interact with. Bjorn is the exception. He is the CT technician who regularly attends to my scans. He does recognise me and knows that I had scans just a month ago, so he would most likely realise that something new has come up. I'm not sure why, but his familiar presence is somewhat reassuring and comforting.

Having a bone scan means that a small amount of radiation is injected, and you wait a couple of hours so it can penetrate your bones before scanning. I met my sisters for lunch in between, and we managed to pass the time without anything too emotional. Family and friends have had years of experience to know that if I wish to discuss cancer, I will, and if not, it's their job to distract.

After the bone scans were completed, it was a waiting game until the results were known the following day. The scan report had come back clear. There is no definitive answer to the lesion in my arm.

It is difficult to put into words the relief. In a way, it is just as forceful as anxiety, but in a good way. I unwind the coil and reverse the direction of the spin. And just like that, stability has returned to my world.

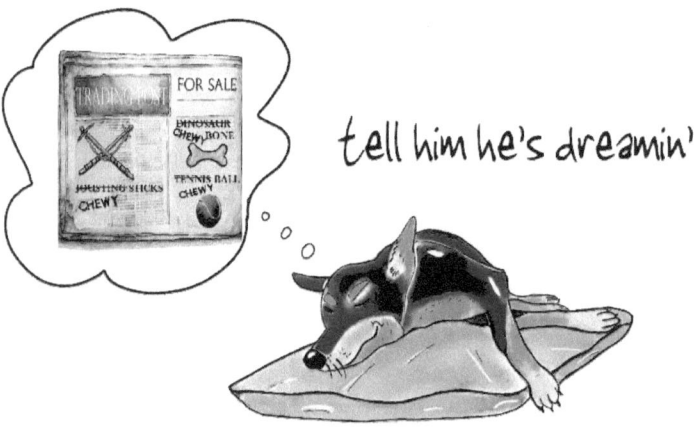

Wednesdays with Harry
GOD SAVE THE QUEEN

September 14, 2022

It's getting late, about 11 pm, and it occurs to me that another sleep-deprived night is ahead…this time by choice. I invited Harry to join me in witnessing this significant moment in history; however, his desire to sleep takes precedence.

Yes, I am becoming drowsy and may periodically droop my head in an involuntary, sleepy motion; however, I cannot draw my attention away too long from the most historical and ceremonial, poignant event currently underway in London.

I realise that watching it 'live' will place it in that small box that holds my memories of such noteworthy and historical moments in time…where only the most important and momentous occasions are allowed to reside. Besides the glorious sporting victories, unfortunately, many of those moments are shrouded in death. I recall a fellow student, Jane Kitto, beside herself with grief when we were on a school trip to Canberra when Elvis passed away. I was up a ladder picking cherries when John Lennon's assassination was announced on my battery-powered trannie and listening to Rex Hunt pause his footy commentary to break the news of Diana's death. So I know that tonight, watching the Queen's coffin in the sombre march towards Westminster Abbey will be well remembered and stored away. But, of course, it is somehow more than that. For me, the infinitesimal price of tiredness is not just about curiosity; it is about paying my own respect to the most amazing woman.

Reverence is seeping out from beyond the broadcast as I watch thousands of heartbroken people lining the streets, witnessing Her Majesty's final journey. The family following her coffin appears stoic, in full ceremonial mind, yet the depth of their sorrow is present.

The sound of silence is only interrupted by the clatter of the disciplined, well-rehearsed military parade. The solemn occasion demands such a ceremony. It is not only what the British are known for and do best, but in this case, is acknowledging their devotion and love for not only the greatest of Monarchs, but also enduring admiration and respect for the woman Elizabeth.

Her military leader leads the march, but it is not just a uniform on display; it is personal. Her coffin is surrounded by her guards, hugging her presence and guiding her safely to rest for one last time.

Since learning of her passing, I have surprised myself with how emotional I have felt. I haven't really considered myself a monarchist, but perhaps I am. I understand the pomp and ceremony, the traditions and extravagant processions are dripping with the impractical and possibly seen as redundant pageantry...But I like it. Much like the reason that I sing 'now bring me some figgy pudding' in full yuletide voice at Christmas – not making any sense, yet fills me with tradition, and an infinite amount of joy.

I realise there are voices believing that now is the appropriate time to question our place in the Commonwealth and those who have reasons to frown upon such a monarchical rule. But now is not the time. Now is the time to give those who grieve space and for the most remarkable woman to be given the farewell she deserves.

I am not sure that future generations will ever come to know such an example of dedicated service to her country and commonwealth, and I feel very privileged to have lived during her reign.

BIGGEST MORNING TEA

> The human brain starts working the moment you are born and never stops until you stand up to speak in public.
> —George Jessel

In my experience, there couldn't be a more accurate quote!

Recently, I was asked to speak at a function for the Cancer Council's Biggest Morning Tea. It was for my parents' retirement village and so armed with the hope that a good cup of tea may distract, and with the expectation that hearing loss may be rife, I cautiously agreed.

My objection to public speaking can also be summed up from this quote from Jerry Seinfeld

'According to most studies, people's number one fear is public speaking. Number two is death. Death is number two. Does that sound right? This means to the average person, if you go to a funeral, you're better off in the casket than doing the eulogy.'

Days leading up to the event meant copious notes taken, bullet points memorised and many rehearsals in front of a mirror. Which, by the way, only seemed to amplify the horrific realisation that my mouth appeared to be working in complete opposition to my brain, which was resulting in muddled verbal dribble.

Of course, I am completely au fait with the subject matter... I have even written a book about it... so what was stopping my confidence from performing for a crowd? Writing allows me the luxury of creating perfectly eloquent and articulate sentences that can be repeatedly edited until the exact message and degree of purpose are met. How can my chemo brain cope with the verbal equivalent?

There were more than a hundred elderly, generous souls in attendance that day, and whilst they looked kind and forgiving, that mindset was immediately put to the test when the microphone spluttered to a stop halfway through my practised opening sentence. Fortunately, a chap named Bert, from the organising committee, was relatively quick to shuffle to my aid. He trundled about in the storeroom for a while and eventually, yet enthusiastically, produced a second microphone. This slight pause in proceedings allowed my anxiety to grow as I stood awkwardly hugging my notes in front of an expectant crowd.

Microphone number two was tested and appeared reliable, and so I began again. Juggling notes, my book, and the microphone, combined with my limited fine motor skills, was indeed a challenge. I then made it through a few minutes until the power cord fell out, and again I came to a stammering stop. Perhaps this was a sign?

Maybe this was a common occurrence, as the seemingly undaunted and undeterred sea of eager faces remained focused in my direction. So, with the realisation that divine intervention was unlikely, I had little option but to take a deep breath, plug the mic back in, and proceed.

Was it the best speech about cancer? Nope. But in the end, I am hopeful that my message about positivity and purpose was enough.

The morning tea then flowed, and they raised over $2000 for the Cancer Council. So, yay. As I was preparing to leave, Bert declared that the use of their lectern may have helped. Yes indeedy!

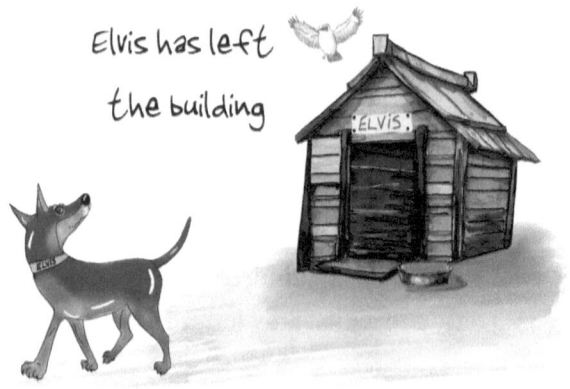

Wednesdays with Harry
PRINCES PIER

Harry actually suggested an activity for today, AND it wasn't sporting related. He proposed we look at the old pier area in Port Melbourne, which attracts many keen photographers. Brilliant, so to Port Melbourne it is, and specifically the Princes Pier.

The Spirit of Tasmania ferry is patiently awaiting her journey across the Bass Strait, and we discuss the possibility of spontaneously escaping to Tasmania. Unfortunately, cancer treatment steals away impulsive liberties. Those carefree days seemed so long ago.

Walking towards the pier, we are enveloped by the sights and smells of the sea. Hungry seagulls hover above, loitering, awaiting to swoop upon any morsel of abandoned sustenance. Fishermen cast their long-reaching lines. Their confident know-how is fused with territorial arrogance, and they are unaware of tangling fishhooks into oblivious passersby. An oil slick slides apart long enough to spy six scarlet starfish and one old, tattered boot nestled on the seabed. The hue of the emerald algae adhered to the rocks is blindingly vivid, and the choice of Harry's ruby red striped socks seems oddly appropriate to counteract the fog that has surrounded our view.

The Railway Pier is no longer workable. The remains of the railway tracks, which signified the railway's purpose when it was built in 1915, are still evident. It was renamed Princes Pier in 1920 when the Prince of Wales (Edward VIII) came to visit. The forest of weathered posts and pylons reach up from the bay, creating rows of wooden sentries; an army standing tired, proud, and defiant. The boards that would have once sat proudly on top are no longer attached. You would think that would render the pier useless, no longer with a purpose or function. It is indeed the opposite. The value of this relic now lies in its quest to be observed. The colours and textures invite you to linger and absorb its history, and I found myself mesmerised.

The fact that I was more content to sit and soak in this scene than when placed in front of some of history's greatest artists at the NGV probably suggests something of my character. Harry's usual pursuit of keeping these activities quick-paced finally surrendered, and he yielded to the pylons' command for attention.

Among the past and the present, the seagulls, the fog and the sounds of the sea, we found solace - and simply sat.

So there you go...

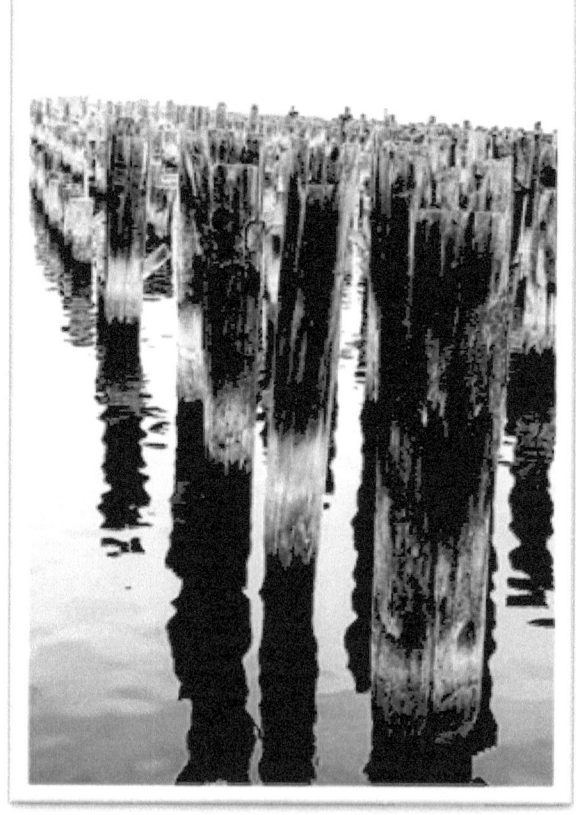

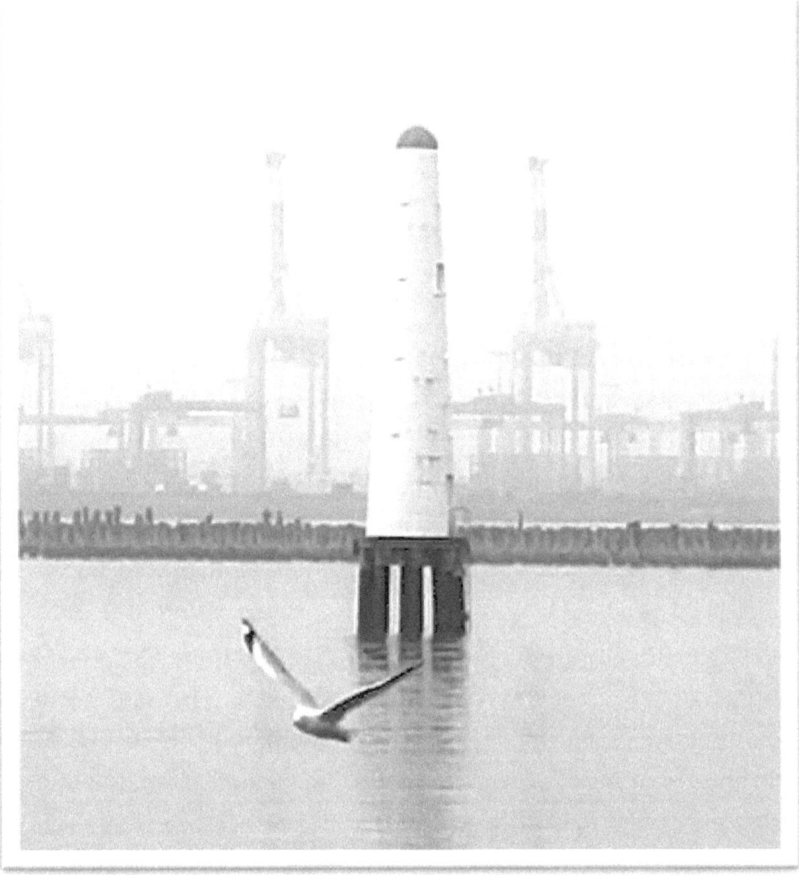

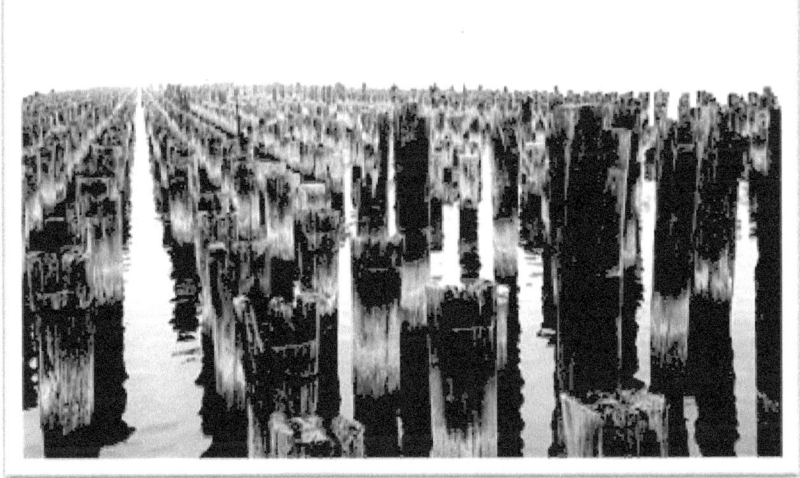

LIVER METS
June 9th to July 24th 2023

Perhaps the following photo of a wardrobe looks quite out of place in this book, but to me, it is so very significant and meaningful.

Five days prior, this wardrobe in Harry's room was painted navy blue to match the life-size poster stickers of former Carlton footballers Brendon Fevola and Chris Judd, which were adhered to the outside. The inside doors housed a collection of stickers representing youth and the need to mark one's territory. From Lego to Vans, Nike, Apple, and Save the Dolphins. I suspect it wasn't a calculated collection, simply one with a single criterion. Lifetime adhesion. I wish I had a 'before' photo because only then can one appreciate the difference five days have made. The sanding, the scraping, the preparing, the precisely cut mitered corners to create the illusion of panels, the undercoating, the painting, and finally the decorating with new knobs.

But this chapter isn't about the carpentry work I completed; it is about what these doors represent. Distraction.

Five weeks prior, I received some pretty difficult news regarding cancer. A routine CT scan revealed that my liver was showing innumerable metastatic lesions. If you are cancer savvy, you will understand that lesions to your liver are a pretty dire situation. I was informed that my only option was to go back onto aggressive chemo, which may buy me a few months.

Here I was, cruising about in the metastatic cancer world, fearlessly declaring I would live forever, and then suddenly I was hit with the most enormous hammer. It's hard to explain the level of anxiety and fear when your life is now measured in months.

You may have already noted that I was in a similar situation a few years ago when I was told the lung nodules had progressed. That turned out to be false, so I knew that I needed additional tests to believe what I was being told was correct. There was a hesitant approach from the medical world to test further, as they felt there was no doubt about the diagnosis and prognosis. It was, however, agreed to follow up with an ultrasound the following week. The result of that showed nothing on my liver. I was told that this was because the lesions were too small for the ultrasound, and while an MRI could be more definitive, as a public patient, I was informed that there was no funding available to cover the cost.

I had a very strong desire to escape, and so Harry and I jumped on a plane and ran away to Tasmania for four days. The gravity of the situation was not lost on Harry, and he really was quite the rock. He shrugged off his youthful coat and truly understood the need to distract, laugh and enjoy this time.

The mental tsunami was threatening, and all hope was hanging by a thread from a phone call. My situation was referred to a multidisciplinary team of oncologists and radiologists to determine if the CT scan report was accurate. I received the news from my oncologists while boarding the ferry from Bruny Island.

The original results stood. No hope was given as they couldn't see that the result could be anything other than liver mets.

I retreated to numbness.

Somewhere in the depths of my being, I still questioned their determination, and so I knew I needed a plan. Regardless of how dire a problem is, having a plan truly helps.

With the support of my GP, I found my own liver specialist, a brilliant liver expert who suggested that hope was not lost and that other outcomes were possible. He then quickly organised an MRI.

I'm unsure if it was a sign, nor why I selected showtunes to listen to, but the allocated headphones during that MRI were playing

Sinatra crooning, 'I did it my way', and Doris Day singing Que Sera Sera!'

A few days later, I was informed that the MRI results were clear and that no lesions were found.

It was five weeks of stress, fear and concern, but I am blessed to have had enormous love and support from a few friends and family. I realise it is not just me who is affected by such news.

To anyone going through the crappity crap of cancer, hold on tight to those closest - and ask for second opinions! Those five weeks taught me to trust my instincts once again, but also to pursue a life with no limitations. I am grateful to be here still and owe it to myself to live a fulfilled life. In these weeks, I learnt to breathe, dabbled with Qi Gong, prayed with monks and listened to countless seminars on healing.

It is alarming that on three occasions now, the progression of cancer mets has been determined and all three times misdiagnosed. It concerns me how often this may happen to those who do not seek further options or opinions.

Whilst the relief was enormous, for a period after, I really did struggle with the associated mental trauma.

These wardrobe doors will always be a reminder that distraction and living in the present are so important….and that stickers take enormous determination to remove!

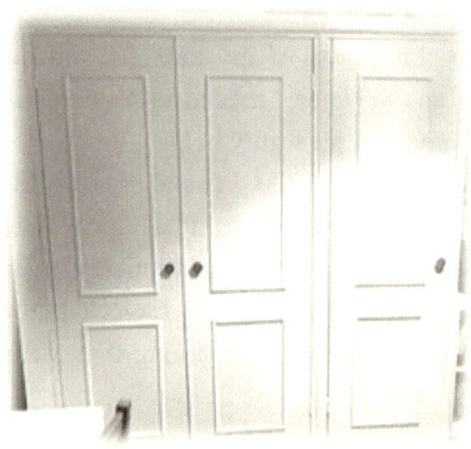

Wednesdays with Harry
GREAT EXPECTATIONS

This morning, I scrutinised the fruit bowl and carefully selected what appeared to be a juicy ripe peach. My anticipation for the succulent taste of summer was quickly and sadly shattered with a familiar feeling of disappointment when I bit into the bruised inner layer. Deception by stone fruit. Of course, when actually purchasing produce, I realise that expecting every piece to be a perfectly formed agricultural miracle is not realistic; however, I live in hope.

I initiated a conversation with Harry on this topic. He strongly believes that having low expectations is the only way to go. He explained that aiming relatively low lessens the chance of dissatisfaction or disappointment. He justified his ideals by citing passing his university exams.

'Mum, if I aim for fifty per cent, that is a pass, and I'll be happy with that, and anything higher is a bonus', he declared.

I, of course, am horrified to think that he is actually only expecting fifty per cent and start to question who has raised him. So, I immediately leap into parent-teaching mode and attempt to reason that low expectations can also lower your standards and, sadly, be satisfied with second best. In contrast, greater expectations create a positive and determined attitude. Then he reminds me of all the football games we have attended with anticipation and high expectations for a win, only to be left traumatised and disillusioned. Well, I think traumatised is a tad dramatic, and I explain that it is character-building and creates resilience. He declares that until Carlton makes the finals, they will remain on his list of low expectations.

Aha, so you have a list! That would suggest that you also have high expectations. I probed him for further information. His list consisted of No, Low, and High expectations. If football and Uni exams were low, then what would he consider high?

After some thought, he declared that he had high expectations that his mother would regularly annoy him with these pointless discussions.

The roll of his eyes suggested that this conversation had peaked and was quickly going to conclude.

My own list of expectations is as follows:

NO EXPECTATIONS:
- That housework is done by others
- That I will get an uninterrupted night's sleep
- That I will win the lottery
- That the diet I start on a Monday will last until Tuesday

LOW EXPECTATIONS:
- That good manners will become popular
- That the aging process will be kind
- That everyone knows the difference between 'your and you're'

HIGH EXPECTATIONS:
- That Carlton will win a flag in this decade
- That Harry will pass his exams
- That all fruit is edible
- That miracles happen
- That I will continue to write nonsense

Now I will go about my day, sweeping the floor whilst only mildly affected by linguistic issues and fully assume that the apple I am about to eat will be delicious!

So there you go...

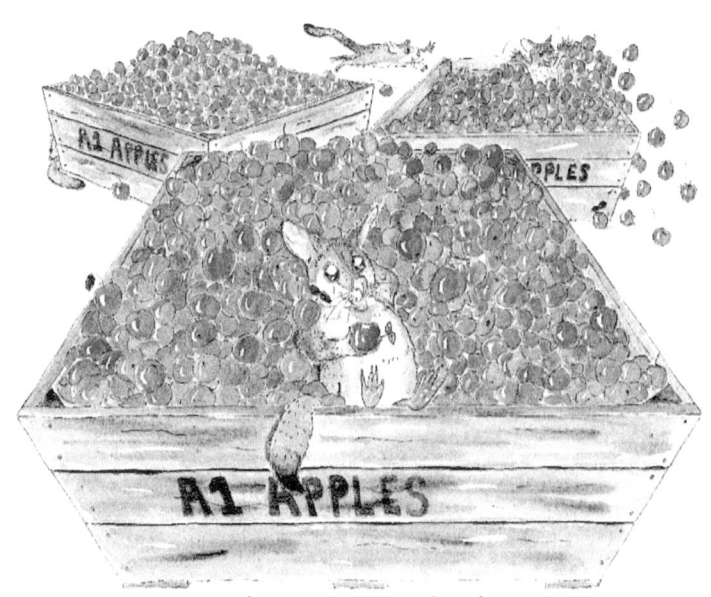

crate expectations

PURPOSE

Many years ago, when I released one of my children's books, *My Melbourne Adventure,* I forwent the usual book launch. Instead, I organised some children's entertainment, roped in family and friends to help, and stormed the Royal Children's Hospital. In cahoots with Captain Starlight, we had a wonderful day donating books to the children and seeing them delighted with entertainment from Carp Productions.

One young boy, who had been in and out of the hospital many times, showed boundless enthusiasm to participate in the interactive production. He had a great time and was the star of the show. A few months later, I received a letter from his grandmother. She explained that he had been quite despondent with his illness and had withdrawn and become generally disinterested. However, since being on stage in the Starlight room that day, he had regained passion in activities and even began attending a drama workshop. She was so thankful for the day we provided. Now I am not kidding myself in believing that I had anything to do with his new zest for life, and if anyone was to be thanked, it was Carp Productions for including him. It was entirely his own will and keenness that led him to engage, but I am so thrilled that I was able to provide a very small stepping stone.

You may never quite know when something you say or do, whether kind or unkind, may influence or affect someone's life.

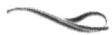

What is your purpose in life? One of those whopping philosophical questions that can leave you pondering late at night, when the noises of the day dissolve and clarity is allowed to prevail. Or perhaps it is contemplated more wisely when you are full of gin and wearing your underwear as a hat. Either way, at some point in our lives, it may crop up.

I would love to have some brilliant and cleverly worded answer that would knock your socks off with admiration and respect. The truth is, however, it is really quite simple.

How does one arrive at a response to such a question? Well, I suppose you first have to want to know that there is an answer. When I am struggling to find a solution, I often find it easier to figure out what I don't want, so here are some random notes I have made on various things in my life that I *don't* want. In no particular order:

I don't want to be one-dimensional

I don't want to lose my sense of humour

I don't want to live in the suburbs

I don't want to eat pumpkin

I don't want to feel sorry for myself

I don't want to be greedy

I don't want to be monotonous

I don't want to be judgemental

I don't want to be dismissive

I don't want to feel empty

I don't want to live in fear

I don't want to be conceited

I don't want to be unkind

I don't want to be a burden

I don't want to be complacent

I don't want to be intolerant

I don't want to be lonely

I don't want to miss Harry's life

I don't want to be forgotten

I don't want to die

I am unsure if this is an accepted strategy or if such a template exists. I hope I will be remembered as someone who had a zest for life and treated you well.

So here it is, albeit brief.

My purpose and values in life are to be the best Mum I can be for Harry, live with passion, pay attention, act with kindness…oh, and laugh plenty.

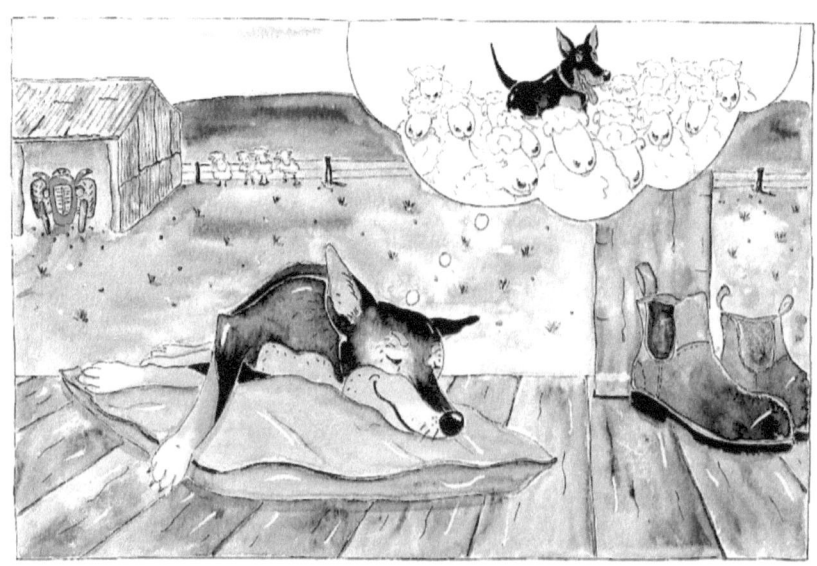

chasing dreams

Wednesdays with Harry
GOLF

For anyone reading the Wednesdays encounters and have concluded and perhaps concerned that Harry is being dragged about to flower shows and town hall tours under hostage like conditions, then worry no more. Today we embarked on the joys – ahem - of golf.

For his birthday last week, Harry's golf bag was adorned with a new putter. This was requested as his last one had broken. I'm not quite sure how a stick of titanium becomes damaged; however, after observing today, I may have a clue!

The deal was that due to the terrain at Warburton golf course, beautiful yet mountainous, I would hire an electric golf cart, puddle about, relax and soak up the gorgeous scenery whilst Harry hit the ball with the sticks. He is actually a pretty good golfer and, on any other day, averages about seven over par. Today, however, was not one of those days.

Firstly, he appeared under pressure from the bloke on the ride-on mower. Where we went, this dude seemed to follow, and I too found myself in a bit of dodgem-style situation on the first, third and fifth fairways. Harry was convinced this renegade ride-on would mow down his ball. He then had to contend with the two talentless nuff-nuffs in front of us who slapped the ball about five metres each hit. We both eventually lost patience, and as they seemed oblivious to the golf etiquette of letting Harry play through, and my usually effective glare was having absolutely no effect, we skipped a hole to zoom past.

Now, I did observe that Harry really can hit the ball well. He was parring many holes and achieving other golfing-term types of outcomes such as *Birdie, Replacing the Divots* and *Addressing the Ball*; however, cracks started to show when I innocently inquired how well his putter was doing. Shooting a seven on a par three when he was on the green in one was the start of the demise. '*Relax,*' I said. '*Look at the gorgeous scenery,*' I advised.

Not a lot of humour in golf, I have discovered.

He did manage to complete the course with all his golf clubs intact. The five-iron and putter appear slightly frightened, but I am sure with a little gentle encouragement, they will recover for future golfing enjoyment!

So there you go…

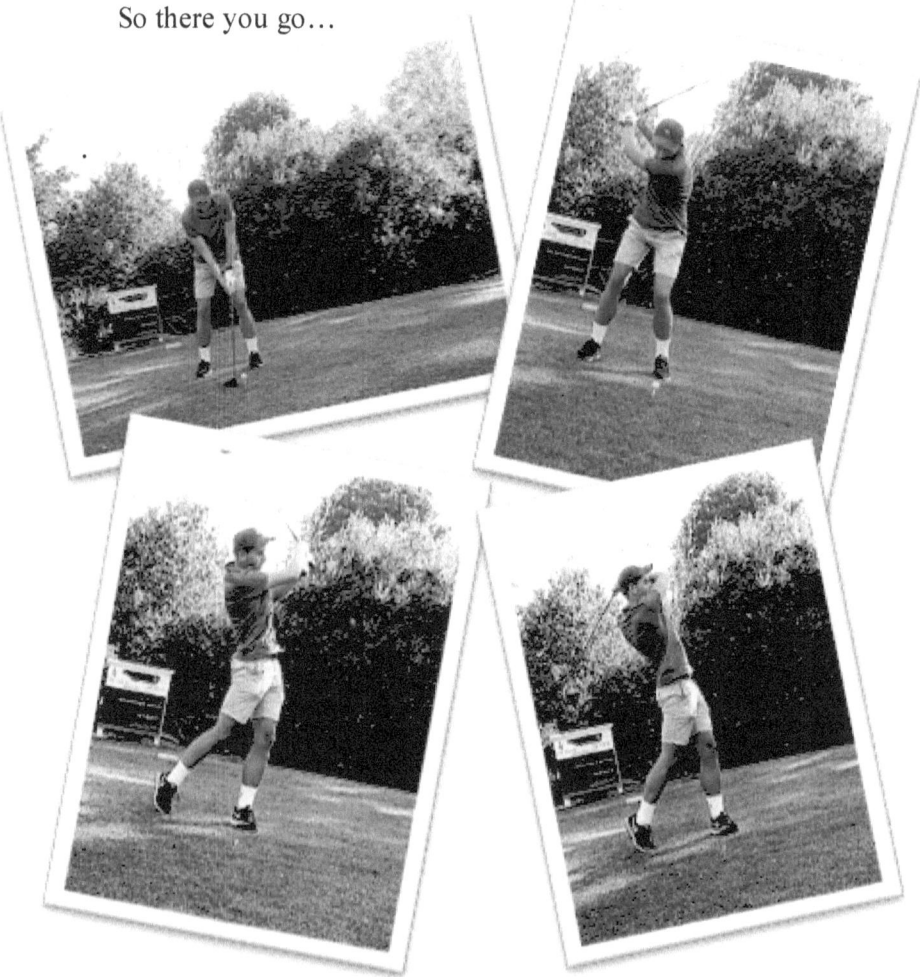

NANETTE

It's one of those days when metastatic cancer smacks me in the face. The dress code for today is dictated by the fact that it is scan day. No metal zips, buckles, buttons, clips or jewellery. That part is easy. The rest, not so much. This day seems to come about too regularly, and whilst I am very familiar with and accept that it is essential, it is a day I have come to dread.

The actual procedures are a tad invasive and inconvenient at best... but it isn't the procedures I dread, but what they signify. The anxious wait for results. It is a period of time when life is on hold until you feel safe to breathe again. The nagging clutter of thoughts that persistently knock about in my mind, and will do for the next five days, until the results are known. Scanxiety is one of those new words, an addition to our language. And just as it should, life goes on around me, oblivious. Distraction is necessary.

I am writing this as I sit in the prep area, waiting for a chest, abdomen, pelvis CT. I have already consumed a copious amount of a contrast drink, not to my taste, I doubt it would be to anyone's taste. The nurses are rejoicing that they managed to locate a suitable vein for a cannula. They recognise me and my elusive veins, and understand that indeed, a first successful attempt is a win.

I was also injected with the radiation necessary for the bone scan later today. I always find it a tad ironic that the staff are gowned, masked, and the injection is housed in a sturdy metal hazchem container for fear of its contents escaping...yet those contents go inside me.

The imaging department is chaotic. Nurses are juggling the initial process and matching paperwork to patients. You cannot help but overhear personal details, including dates of birth and procedure details, being repeated. One woman looks flustered. She was running late as she had mistakenly gone to the breast clinic instead. She needed a biopsy, and I could easily imagine how she might feel. The variety of reasons someone would come to radiology is, of course, vast.

A technician reading a clipboard announces that they are ready for Nanette. Nanette doesn't answer. He repeats her name and looks at me with a hopeful glance, as if I may have perhaps forgotten that my name is Nanette. I shake my head slightly to let him know I am not Nanette. He rushes off to another area, and the echo of his cry for Nanette continues.

It has been an hour since drinking the contrast, so I will likely be next. I start to visualise that my body is healthy and cancer-free.

My name is called, must go...take a deep breath and hold it...

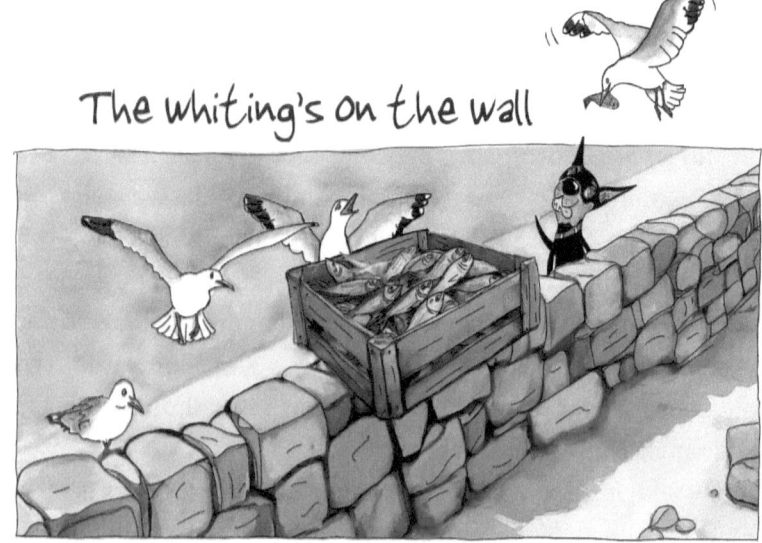

The whiting's on the wall

Wednesdays with Harry
MULLIGAN

A football injury from week one of Harry's season has meant that any spare time this week was spent seeking treatment at the physiotherapist. He appears to have injured his groin. My suggestion to ice the area was initially met with hostility. Once he realised that he needed to move again, he diligently started some rehab.

As a female, it is always a bit of a mystery how blokes manage pain and illness. From witnessing dying carcasses who are couch ridden with the man-flu, to the intense profanity from stubbing a toe. Harry assured me that there was no way that I could possibly know or understand how bad this particular pain was. Of course not. There was very little point in detailing the pain from giving birth to a 4.5kg child, having a breast removed or experiencing a burst appendix! Now, while I realised he was indeed suffering and I applied the appropriate amount of sympathy and compassion, it did become apparent that this pain was being conveniently used to accommodate his own particular agenda. Seemingly, this injury prevented him from doing the dishes, emptying the rubbish and tidying his room. It also became apparent that merely the act of thinking enhanced this unbearable ache, as his University studies were put aside and replaced by educational Seinfeld reruns. Fortunately, after a scan cleared him of any damage and the next football match is fast approaching, the pain has dissipated to a dull twinge. Welcome back Harry.

So we have made it to the Easter break, and whilst I still need to do my end of quarter tax, market some products, write a kids' book, fix the leaky tap, tidy the Tupperware cupboard, clean the bathroom, sew on a button and organize dinner, I have put on the pause button in order to indulge in the glorious warmth of the Autumn sun on my sleepy head.

I am so fortunate to have magnificent scenic views from our backyard. Surrounded by mountains, scarlet, fiery autumnal leaves and sleeping dogs. Ahh, bliss.

Five minutes later, the peace was shattered as our golden retriever, Mulligan, decided it was too hot for her hairy body and so took a quick dip in the doggy pool. I have to say that her pool etiquette is lacking. Her desire to dig and bite at the now swirling whirlpool creates a cascade of water flowing over the edge. Reaching maximum waterlogged capacity, she bounds joyfully and excitedly as close to my dozing self as possible before shaking her water storage entirely over me. Now she is up and about, she may as well find a ball and leap her wet, soggy and hefty self on top of me in an attempt to encourage a ball game. Her keenness to play fetch is somewhat compromised because she refuses to release her jaws from the ball. The struggle to remove the saliva-covered ball from her was quickly waning from my point of view. Alas, Mulligan was still desperately keen. After she relaxed enough for me to pry it off her, and then throw it a ridiculously short distance, she looked at me with utter disappointment and then gave up.

We all settled back into a sunning doze – at least I thought we did. Five minutes later, the peace was shattered as Mulligan decided it was too hot for her hairy body and so took a quick dip in the doggy pool.

So there you go...

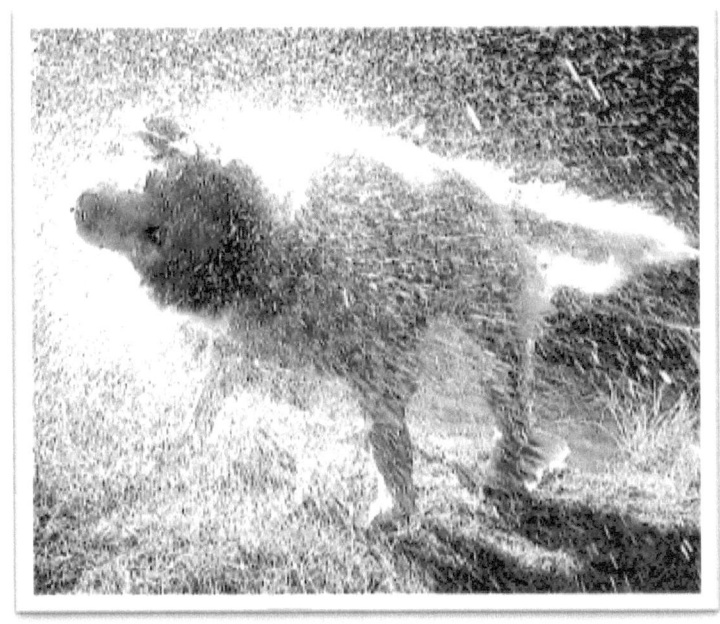

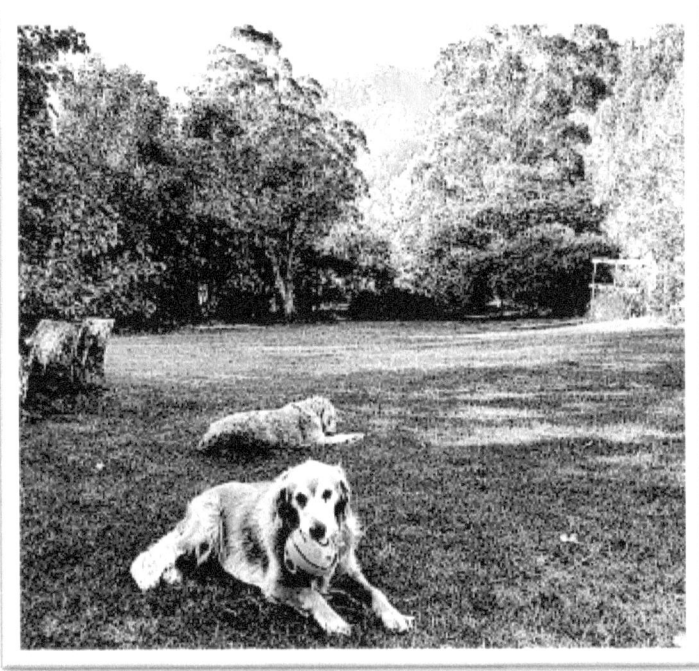

DEAR HARRY

Dear Harry,

There is no doubt you will realise that simply by writing this letter to you will have opened a deluge of emotive sensibilities from me. I know you will be cringing in anticipation of any exaggerated soppiness. Sentiment is not really your thing. It is not that you don't feel emotion or understand sentiment; it's just that you tend to live in the here and now. That is not a bad thing. Your outlook on life is perhaps more complex than you would like others to believe. You want to create the perception that you are laid-back, calm, and not stressed—quite a distance from where you were in your youth. You often point out that there isn't a lot going on in your head of an in-depth nature. I know this isn't always the case. I hope you will eventually trust that experiencing pain can also allow your heart to thrive. If nothing else, life should be about feelings.

I know that all this cancer nonsense hasn't been easy on you. It's pretty overwhelming to think that cancer has been present in our household for more than half of your life. Many times, plans and activities were compromised, and you have had to witness me ill on so many occasions. I can only hope that you are not too mentally scarred and that my dark times have not infiltrated your innocence and outlook on how great life can actually be. I love that in more recent times, when I feel uncertain and question my outcome, you state pretty emphatically and pragmatically, *'you'll be right, Mum, you're going to be okay.'* I'm not sure where you find that confidence and faith, but I'm so glad you do. Never doubt the strength of trust and reassurance.

When you were young, you were convinced that I was magical and knew everything…possibly because I used to tell you that! Fortunately, the problems faced at that age were solvable, and I could live up to the hype. I had all the answers. Eventually, you outgrew that notion, and I no longer sit upon that lofty pedestal. But that is just as it should be. You have outstretched your wings and are fluttering them into independence. I am so proud of all your achievements and efforts. You may not trust me enough to cut your hair during the lockdown in Covid, no matter how boofy it looks, but I do hope you still trust me enough to know that I am always here for you. No matter what.

There is a well-known poem called **'I wish you enough' by Bob Perks**

Now don't groan, but here is my version, just for you.

Harry,

I wish you enough kindness to warm your heart,

I wish you enough strength to handle the crappy stuff,

I wish you enough happiness to brighten your soul,

I wish you enough sorrow to know the difference,

I wish you enough music for gleeful delight,

I wish you enough curiosity to never be bored,

I wish you enough confidence to take on the world,

I wish you enough gratitude to be forever fulfilled,

I wish you enough resilience to keep barracking for Carlton,

I wish you enough laughter to illuminate your days,

I wish you enough honesty to always be true,

I wish you enough respect to appreciate differences,

I wish you enough good manners - just because,

I wish you enough trust to never despair,

I wish you enough humour to forever be saved,

I wish you enough faith to always believe,

I wish you enough humility to never be arrogant,

I wish you enough dance to feel joy and feel free,

I wish you enough pride to not settle for less,

I wish you enough true friends to never be lonely,

I wish you enough passion for decorating life,

I wish you enough smiles to outshine the dark,

I wish you enough purpose to always find clarity,

I wish you enough love to have and to hold,

I wish you enough.

None of us knows how long we have in this life, and even though challenges have been many and not easy, I hope you will always seek to find a solution. I love you more than I can say, and I always will. You are an extraordinary person, Harry Rothwell, and no matter what the future holds, I will always be your biggest fan.

Love always,
Mum xx

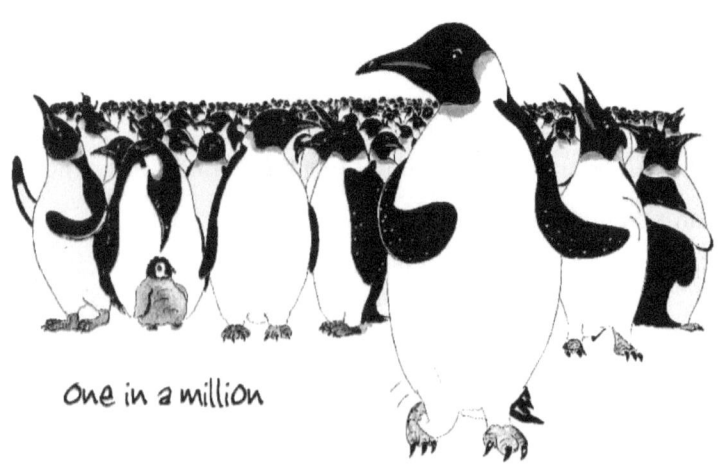

One in a million

Wednesdays with Harry
HONOUR THE MEMORIES

Bit of a slower day today, which suited me just fine. The Botanical Gardens were beckoning for a stroll and a bite to eat; however, like many of our outings, the morning became problematic. After Harry eventually dragged himself out of slumber, he decided that a two-hour run was what he needed to start the day. I absolutely admire his commitment to fitness, even if it does mean that lunch is pushed back to mid-afternoon.

Joining us in the outdoor cafe area were various other late lunch-goers; hundreds of Indian Mynas ready to swoop on the unsuspected discarded crumb; and the piercing yelp from a very yappy dog.

A couple sitting close by were sipping their wine, seemingly oblivious to the noise their Cocker Spaniel was creating, having tied it up around the corner. It was clear that other lunch-goers were jointly focusing annoyance and displeasure in their direction. Heads were turning, and faces were clouded; however, the couple remained steadfast in their plan to finish their smashed avo on sourdough and glass of pinot. I thought it prudent to assist and so unleashed my glare. Now it may just be that the timing of my glare coincided with the completion of their meal, but either way, they downed their drinks, retrieved their pet and went on their way. I do believe that our fellow lunch-goers were quietly applauding my glare ability.

The opportunity to partake in a gondola-type activity and be punted around the lake was located near the cafe, complete with a gondolier, boat hats, and a parasol. Visions of reproducing a Monet watercolour came rushing into my mind. *'Fantastic!'* I enthusiastically declared. Alas. With chest puffed up to suitably express his objection, Harry announced that not in his lifetime would he participate in any parasol and boat hat activity. So, I gave up the notion, and we went for a walk instead.

Providing the opportunity to rest and perhaps gain contemplative reflection is clearly a priority here at the Botanical Gardens. Scattered haphazardly or, indeed, strategically, is a vast array of park benches. Many of these seats have been honoured with inscriptions from loved ones. I decided our task would be to try to find as many memorial plaques as possible. And there were many. Harry failed to understand the need to read the engravings and declared that the actual use for a park bench was for lying on and taking a nap. Of course.

I think it is quite brilliant that these everlasting dedications to loved ones exist. They are not only sentimental tributes to loving memories, but for a brief moment, they allow us to step inside and imagine their lives.

Perhaps someone will honour me like that one day – although hopefully not too soon.

So there you go…

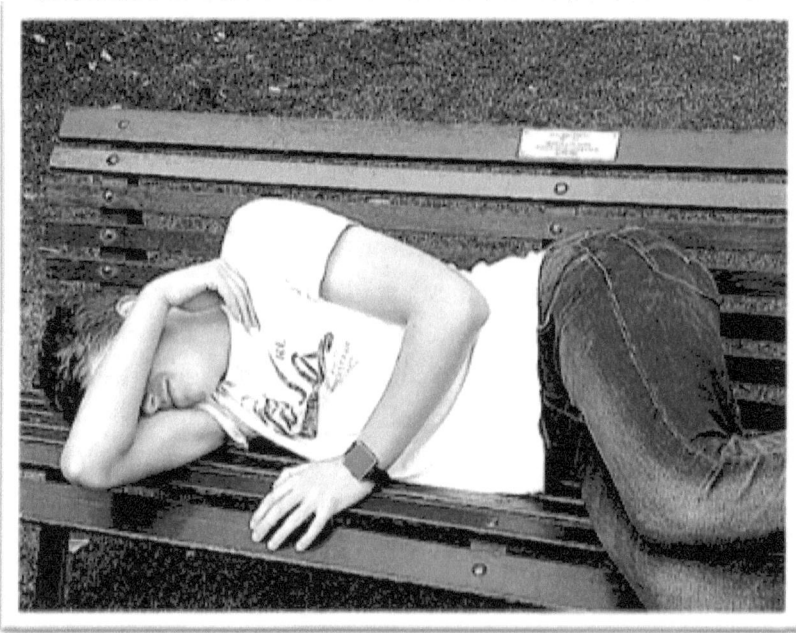

THEM'S FIGHTIN' WORDS

Over the years, I have heard the words *fighting* and *battling* cancer often. I understand why these words are used, but I choose not to use them myself. Enduring and tolerating is perhaps more appropriate. I deliberately avoid encouraging an aggressive war that invades my headspace.

It may feel appropriate to be against an enemy and believe you are showing strength. But what does that say if you die? Do you lose the fight? Did you fail? Is there something you did or didn't do that affected the outcome? Were you not strong enough, not resilient enough? Of course not.

I think there is an appropriate time for these combative words, and if you are honest, you will know when that will be.

I completely understand why those close to you may use such lingo. There is frustration and anger because you cannot control the outcome, and giving cancer the face of an enemy is a natural response. But I believe that if I invite these words to define my dealings with cancer, then I am declaring a war that I will not win. I choose to totally diminish any power that may be bestowed upon cancer. I suffocate its image by treating it with tolerance and acceptance. Hating cancer is simply detrimental to my health.

If we are going to talk about fighting cancer, then let's start with fighting to find a cure. That is truly the only fight that is really going to count in the end.

Perhaps this is as good a place as any to publicly declare that when my life has ended, please don't say she '*fought*' or '*battled*' cancer. Mention my love for my son, family, friends and dogs, sense of humour, love of travelling and writing, and desire to win at Pictionary...but please don't mention cancer. It simply isn't worthy.

Wednesdays with Harry
AFTERMATH
January 4th, 2024

I'm not quite sure if there's an official day for packing away Christmas, but as hot cross buns are already on sale in Coles, I figure today is acceptable. I encourage Harry to partake in this necessary task, but his less-than-enthusiastic contribution in tugging delicate ornaments off the tree ensures that I will take over and let him go back to watching the cricket.

I too love watching the cricket, so, in between uttering a few expletives at Australia's batting performance, I untangled the baubles from the tree, think twice about organising the lights, carefully wrapped the snow globes, dragged the tree outside, vacuumed the pine needles and rearranged the furniture.

Ultimately, I found a few untagged gifts that were left lonely and unwanted under the tree. These are the pressies that are purchased because you wandered into the Christmas section of a department store and succumbed to the ornate and elaborate packaging. At the time, it seemed inconsequential as to who would benefit from lavender-infused preserved figs and caramelised wattle seed pretzels. With no clue as to who would enjoy such treats, these purchases then become backup gifts. Their only function is to remain wrapped and sit under the tree...just in case. Just in case someone pops in unexpectedly, you can enthusiastically offer them one of these well-considered gifts. The question then remains as to how long they sit in stoic preparation. Most likely until Aunty Mildred drops in or until I completely forget what I bought and then joyfully unwrap with delightful anticipation.

Every year, usually sometime in February, I discover a random decoration that has escaped my notice. Eventually, I will have unintentionally created Christmas all year round!

Clearly though, I now need to move the now bauble-free tree from outside the kitchen. In only a matter of four hours since denuding it, I have startled myself at least three times thinking some hairy git is peering in the window! Now, back to the cricket.

So there you go…

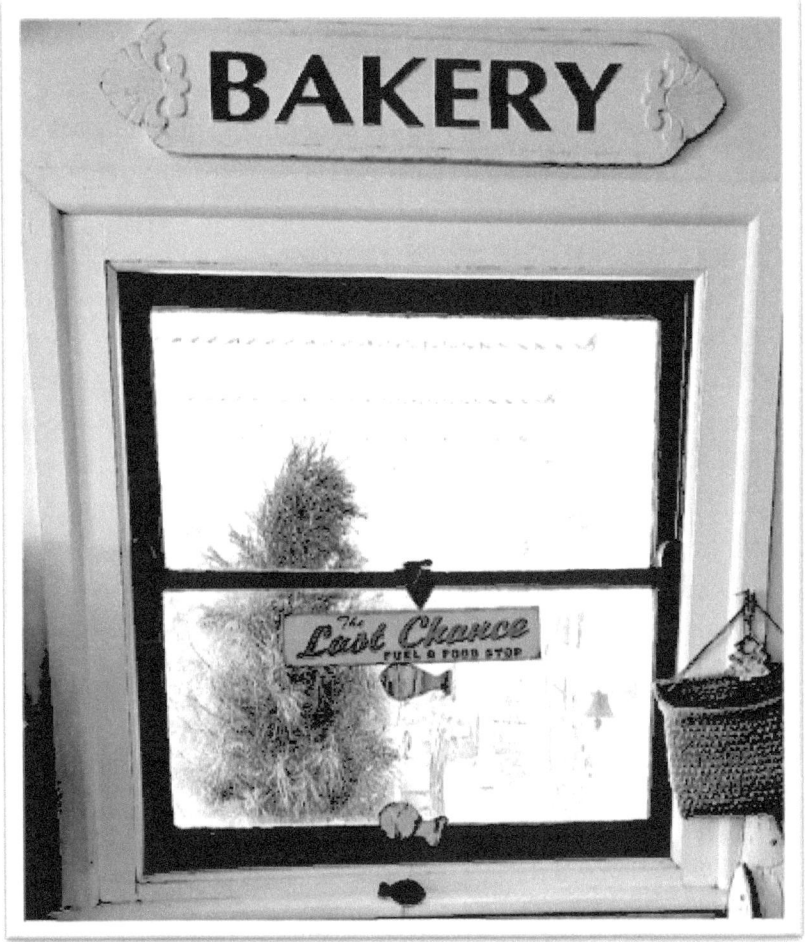

DEBBIE

January 25th, 2024

The wave of emotion that rattled my day, of course, was completely valid. Today, I attended the funeral of a friend.

On the drive to the crematorium, my mind was filled with a mixture of apprehension and sadness. Apprehension of the outpouring of grief that has and would await, and how I would react. Sadness for the finality of a life that was stolen away.

For a while, I was distracted, and my emotions shifted to annoyance as I was stuck driving behind a small white hatchback that was moving excruciatingly slowly. The driver didn't appear to understand that I couldn't be late for a funeral. I then turned on my Spotify playlist to ease my overreaction. It is quite an eclectic combination of music that shuffles from Dire Straits to The Pogues without concern. The melancholy, haunting tune 'Over the Rainbow' is Eva Cassidy's contribution, and I cannot help but be overcome by emotion. It's tempting to flick 'next'. But I don't. I stick with it and allow my feelings to go there. Little did I know then that Eva Cassidy would be included later in the service. I arrived at the crematorium with enough time to spare.

I knew Debbie from high school — a million years ago — and after that, we had occasional catch-ups but mainly reconnected via social media. That connection grew stronger this past year, which is sometimes inevitable when the cancer circle tightens. For Debbie it was brain cancer and the crappiest one at that. It hit and destroyed in just over a year. Ultimately, I knew that there was nothing I could do that could genuinely help.

The overflow of mourners at the funeral was a solid indication of the love and respect that Debbie deserved. Her gregarious personality, family-oriented nature, community-mindedness, and vivacious qualities reached far and wide. The feeling of grief and perhaps also disbelief was evident. The minister conducting the service gave reassurance that, on this day of all days, it was okay to let go of that emotion.

I was aware that my friendship was more peripheral than others, and the level of emotion would perhaps reflect that. Regardless, the emotion did flow when her children and her brother bravely and tearfully battled their way through the eulogy.

Halfway through, I arrived at that cross-section. That is where I have to decide whether to truly listen and be led uncontrolled by the emotional tributes or stare at the bird in the picture to the right of me in the hope that distraction will hold back the tide. I chose to listen.

It is easy to place ourselves in someone's story and imagine what it would be like if this were our own. While similarities may be present, it isn't the case. The only place I need to put myself today is in thought and tribute to Debbie.

After the service, many followed the hearse to Deb's final place of rest. The fascination and curiosity of her grandchildren regarding the depth of the grave that had been dug allowed for a lighter moment, and mourners were able to engage in small talk before the reality of the situation once again loomed.

I watch as the funeral staff offer necessary instructions to the pallbearers on how to carry and lower her casket onto the pulley system that hovers above her grave. I did find myself wondering if there could be a more efficient and less precarious method.

The minister resumes and speaks the final poignant words of committal. For a brief moment, this group of people surrounding Debbie are of one. More tears are shed as Eva Cassidy's rendition of 'Over the Rainbow' is played, and finality is realised.

Like many mournful situations, we are not built to endure such heavy sorrow. We take a deep breath and begin the journey of figuring out how this particular sadness will fit into our lives.

I am glad I could attend the tribute and celebration of Debbie's life today, and I realise that my sadness is inconsequential compared to her family and her close friends and that my life will continue seemingly unscathed. But it isn't. It is scathed in the knowledge that Debbie's life was cut short because of a hideous disease, and it is scathed for the hurt that will be felt by so many.

Today, my world briefly came to a standstill to pay tribute. Tomorrow, I will continue to do what I do and carry the loss.

I don't know exactly when, or how often you will come into my mind, but I do know that the next time Eva Cassidy pops up on my playlist, I will smile…or maybe cry… either way, I will remember you, Debbie Sadlier. R.I.P.

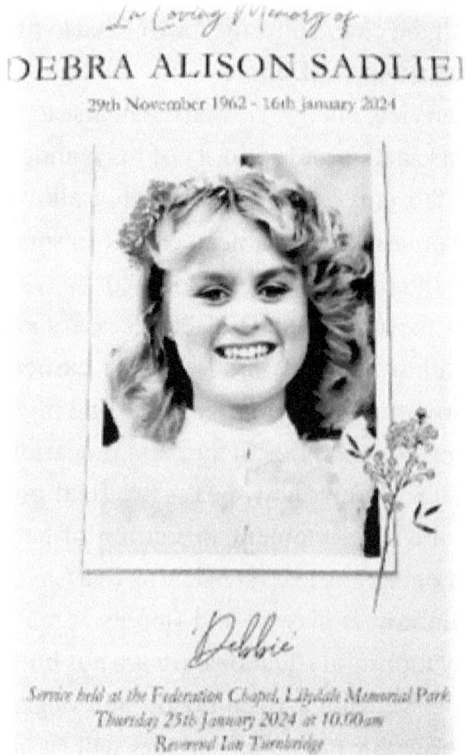

Wednesdays with Harry
GRADUATION

Alarm set for 4.55 am, but in reality, my annoyingly inbuilt mental alarm alerted me at 1.30, 3.30, and Mulligan managed to nudge me awake at 4.30 am, so the fear of sleeping past my actual alarm was completely unwarranted. These types of mornings require precise movements to walk out the door at the allocated time. Besides the slight resistance from my contact lenses, I did manage to switch the motor on at precisely 5.25 am.

In the early hours, I assumed the roads would be free of traffic and we could amble along to our destination, some two hours away, without any concerns. I assumed wrong. I found myself dancing with every type of ute and tradie van, driven by the enthusiastically determined, who all seemed to adopt the notion that speed limits in the early morning were simply a suggestion.

BUT…today was not about traffic or early morning issues…today was all about Harry and the past six years studying at Deakin University. The stress of assignments, essays, exams, word count, practicals, internships and HECS fees was now a mere memory (well, clearly not yet the HECS), as today Harry graduated…not one, but two degrees. A Bachelor of Sports Science and Exercise and a Bachelor of Business (Sports Management).

Today was about dressing the part, cap and gown in place, seated in an auditorium among hundreds of worthy fellow students, academics seated on stage with resident faculty adding glorious colours in their ceremonial attire. Speeches were made and futures discussed as we all witnessed the event with the utmost pride. The only stress was understanding when it was my turn to capture Harry's stage appearance on film, that, and a slight concern that the mashed banana squashed onto my seat by the toddler sitting next to me would emulsify into my shirt.

There were tears of immense pride and smiles of utter joy. Pride in Harry's determination to complete his degrees, even when the struggle was evident. Pride that he has grown into a man who is taking on every opportunity that comes his way.

So, that was today – okay, the trip home from Geelong, yes, Geelong!- was yet another traffically-challenging trip, resulting in a few more expletives, but there you go.

The honour of witnessing today will be forever cherished.

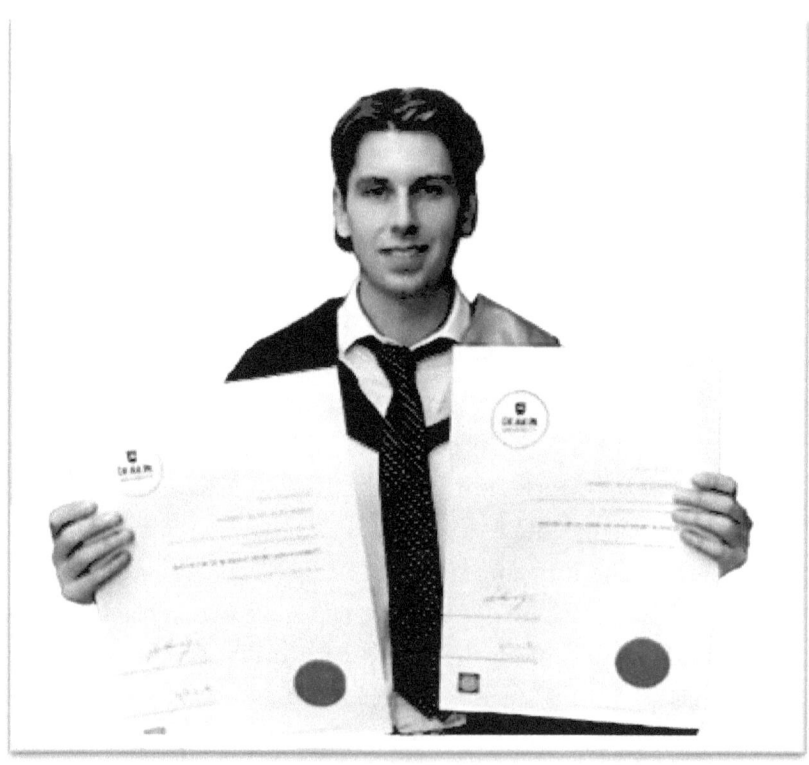

TOMORROW NEVER DIES

Whilst this is the last chapter in this book, I feel confident that it is far from the last chapter of my life. When I look back to 2011, when first diagnosed with cancer, I can clearly see that so many changes have occurred and know that it really is your choice how you respond or react to whatever is thrown your way.

In the early '80s, I regularly caught the train from Lilydale to and from work in the city. It is unlikely you will be aware of the various carriages used during that period if you are younger than forty. There were the shiny new silver trains, the older blue ones and the ancient red rattlers. The blue trains and red rattlers didn't have automated closing doors, which meant that any last-minute, desperate passenger could franticly jump on board as the train pulled out from the station. Their carriages were divided into compartments, and facing each other were bench seats with room to seat three passengers. There were high windowed partitions between sets of seats.

One sweltering summer day, I was sitting on the end of the bench seat, and directly opposite was an elderly woman. Next to her was a vacant seat with a young bloke sitting on the far right-hand side. The whistle had blown, *mind the gap* had been broadcast, and the train began to pull away from Camberwell station. With the doors still widely ajar, a briefcase-carrying, suit-wearing businessman type bloke leapt into the moving train and went to sit in the vacant middle seat opposite. The momentum of the train pushed against him, and he lost his balance. To stop his fall, he reached to brace himself on the partition window that separated the compartments. Unfortunately for all involved, the actual glass from the window was missing, which resulted in his hand gripping and pressing onto the back of a bloke's head seated on the other side. The train gathered speed, and because he was leaning forward in the opposite direction, he was left helplessly flailing in this awkward and uncompromising position. Meanwhile, his nose was now almost touching the older woman's face, and his briefcase had flung off and hit the young dude who was seated to his right. I realise that I could have possibly tried to assist, but I was laughing too hard to be of any use at all.

You will have noticed the numerous anecdotal accounts that appear throughout this book. I thought I should use this last one to illustrate the differences in reactions.

Of course, individual responses are all relevant to your own involvement and perception of the situation. In this case, the businessman was mortified and apologetic; the bloke whose head was being used as a ballast was angry; the older woman looked embarrassed; the young dude was annoyed, and I was crying with laughter. Others witnessing this calamity also had various reactions. Some were concerned, some laughed aloud, some disguised their chuckles behind newspapers, some pretended to sleep, and others turned away. You will be pleased to know that he gave one last big push off the head, regained his balance and finally slinked into the unoccupied seat.

When I recall this incident, I still think it is pretty hilarious. I explained this scenario to Harry. He didn't think it was at all amusing, as just last week, whilst travelling on a train, a middle-aged woman fell into his lap.

The upshot is that I have a choice on how I react to anything in my life.

As far as cancer goes, well, I am very aware that having a chronic illness can become quite one-dimensional. As much as I attempt to dodge the cancer spotlight, I dread that I will eventually become monotonous and tedious to those around me. The topic of cancer is the elephant in the room, and it is the source of great sympathy, empathy, and pity. The truth is, I am not the life of the party anymore, and as much as I wish that it doesn't occupy my life, physically, I am reminded every day. The pragmatist recognises that whilst these side effects are unfortunate, *'you are still alive, so it is better than the alternative'*.

I can cope with the physical effects, but they contribute to a lack of confidence. They are a niggling reminder that my vitality and enthusiasm for life is being tested.

Before the cancer was categorised as *'incurable'*, my view on this whole nightmare differed from what it is now. I understood the various types of cancers, the colours we label them, the honour in surviving, the camaraderie, the significance of milestones, and the attention that comes your way. I wore scarves and hats for comfort and was aware of what that represented.

Now it is very different. Except for the blatantly conflicting fact that I am writing this book, I generally choose to remain incognito. It is a relief to be seen as healthy, part of a larger community that is not dominated by cancer. I now embrace the word *positive*; in fact, I encourage it. Of course, I need to be positive. It is my lifeline, my strength and my hope.

So, with the optimistic expectation that you can cope with yet another list, here are some of what I have learnt:

That my instincts are worth listening to

That I am unique, with individual prognosis and outcomes

That I can have hopes for the future

That Mindfulness is key

That I can choose my reactions

That form is more fun than function

That self-awareness is vital

That the best view is right from my own backyard

That my handwriting is illegible

That I will always struggle with opening bags in supermarkets

That there is no such thing as false hope

That I am not a victim

That Carlton will eventually win

That I still don't like pumpkin

That anger isn't me

That I will always love dogs over cats

That Harry will be okay

That thoughts cannot hurt me

That facing mortality is lonely

That fighting cancer means finding a cure

That advanced cancer is a bit crap

That life will go on, with or without me

That humour is my saviour

That the love of family and friends is imperative

That Wednesdays are a gift

That nurses are angels

That lists are invaluable

That life should be lived

That tomorrow never dies

That I will always be anxious about test results

That I smile often

That when we are no longer able to change a situation, we are challenged to change ourselves.

That I am not dying of cancer, nor living with cancer - I am simply living.

And finally…When the night puts on its cloak, I can choose to dance till dawn.

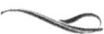

If you have made it to the end of this book, I hope that you will have gained some insights into my experience with cancer, yet appreciate that everyone travels their own path. I know that it helps me to try and diminish the power of cancer, and by succeeding in that narrative, I can live my best life. I don't know what lies ahead for me, but I do know living with hope is my greatest weapon. Ultimately, I also hope that you conclude that this book is more about life than about a disease.

I will continue to go about my day, trying my hardest to live by chasing normal.

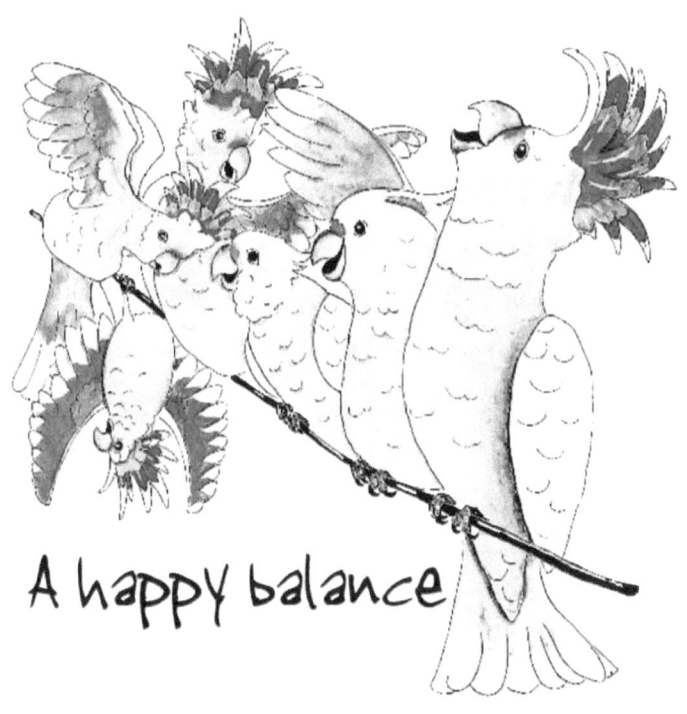

A happy balance

Acknowledgements:

Sincere thanks to all who have encouraged and supported this project. Special nod to Penny O'Brien, Annette Keppel, Leanne Gniel, Pip Young, Gai Basso, Lynne Dwyer, Bryce Rothwell, Jean and Alan Espie, (Mum and Dad) and Harry Rothwell for generously adding your thoughts and emotions.

Genuine gratitude goes to the poor, hand-selected souls I sought to read the first, second, third and twentieth drafts. Including; David Parkin, Celia Burrell, Matthew Knight, Paul Hyndman, Gai Basso, Matthew Pearce, Janet Feher, Kerry Alderuccio, and Pip Young. I sincerely value your feedback and, taking it all into consideration, have primed and preened to finally arrive at satisfaction. Kerry, Pip and Celia – grateful for your additional advice and assistance.

Deep appreciation to all who have gone before and paved the way; sharing stories, fundraising, educating and ensuring advances in cancer treatments are improved. Check out www.loveyoursister.org to learn of ways you can also help.

Eradicating terminal illnesses will eventually be mankind's most remarkable feat.

Look out for further books and other creative products from
Rothwell Publishing: www.rothwellpublishing.com
www.australianadventurepassport.com

www.ingramcontent.com/pod-product-compliance
Lightning Source LLC
Chambersburg PA
CBHW020340010526
44119CB00048B/539